Short Stories for Seniors

105 Large Print, Funny, Engaging Stories Across the Decades

1940 Through 2020; Good Memories to Keep Your Mind Active

Mitchell Bradford Publishing

Table of Contents

Introduction

Welcome to a delightful collection of short stories designed to tickle your funny bone and stir the memories of growing up over the years. These easy-to-read tales are perfect for keeping your mind sharp, sparking conversations, or letting the kids and grandkids read to you for a change.

With large print and bite-sized chapters, this book fits seamlessly into your busy day—whether you're sneaking in a quick laugh or sharing a glimpse of the good old days with younger generations. So sit back, chuckle, and let these stories bring a little joy to your day!

The 1940s

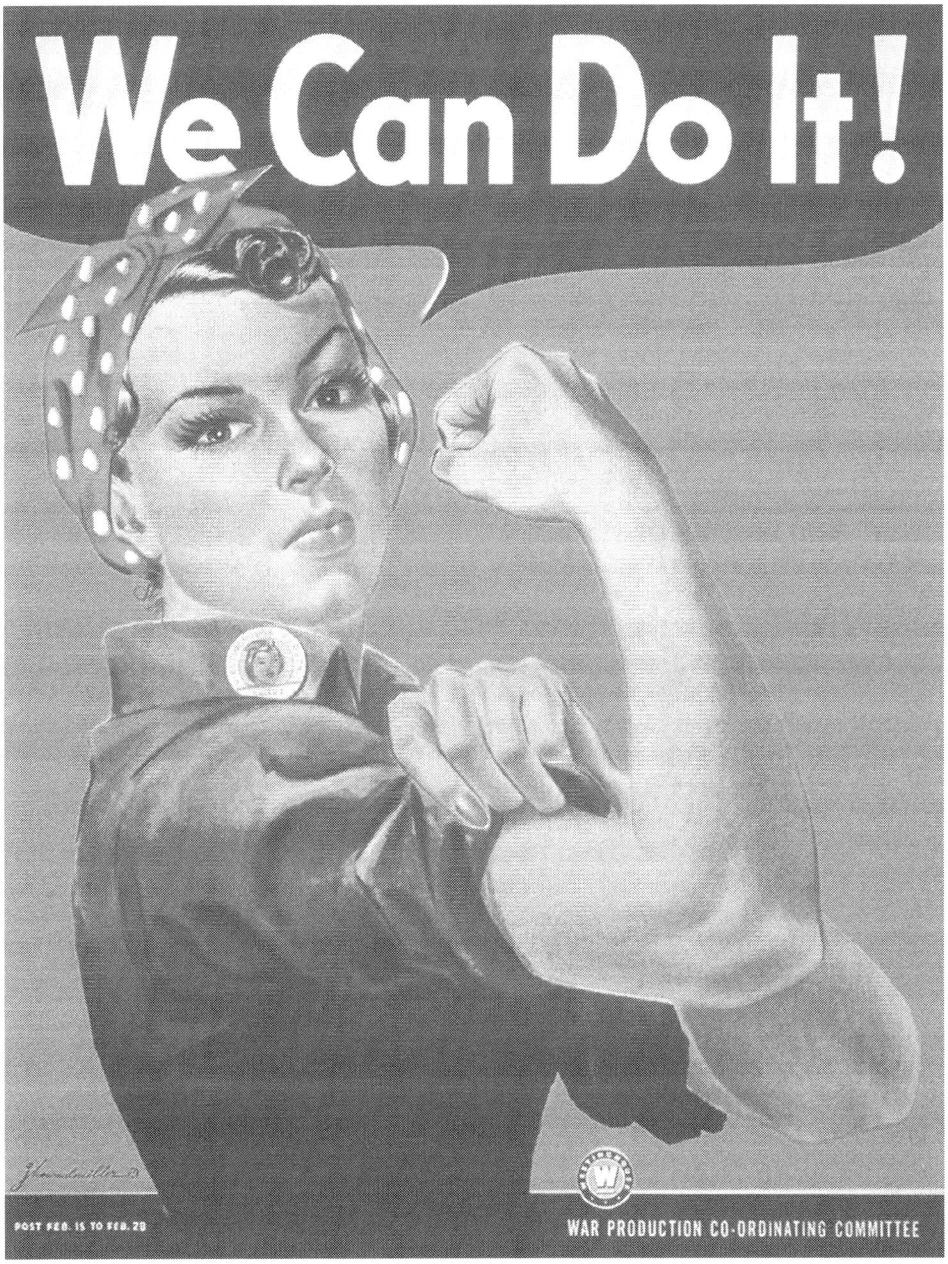
We Can Do It!
POST FEB. 15 TO FEB. 28
WAR PRODUCTION CO-ORDINATING COMMITTEE

Whose Radio Is It?

In 1946, the Marshall family had one prized possession: a big, clunky radio that sat proudly in the living room. It was the heart of the household, providing music, news, and radio dramas that everyone adored. But with only one radio and wildly different tastes, most evenings turned into a battle over what station to listen to.

One Saturday night, the conflict was especially fierce. Mr. Marshall wanted to listen to the news. "There's important stuff happening in the world, and I need to hear it!" he declared, clinging onto the dial like a hawk gripping its prey.

Mrs. Marshall had other ideas. "Oh no, you don't! *The Soap Suds Show* is on! I've been waiting all week to find out if Barbara's long-lost twin is really alive! Your 'stuff' will keep."

The kids, Davey and Betsy, weren't about to sit by quietly. Davey pushed forward. "But, Dad! *The Super Spy Adventures* is about to start! Agent Thompson will catch the bad guy tonight for sure!"

Betsy chimed in, determined not to be left out. "You can't make me miss *Songs for Sweethearts*! They're going to play my favorite tune!"

Davey scoffed. "You say that for all their tunes!"

And so the great Battle of the Radio began. Mr. Marshall twisted the knob to the news. Mrs. Marshall slapped his hand away and cranked it toward her soap opera. Davey reached over both of them, switching it to the spy show, only for Betsy to dart in and spin it to the music station. And the cycle repeated, with fatigue slowly setting in like it was the trenches of 1916 all over again.

This time, though, Spot, the family dog, jumped onto the radio table in all the excitement, knocking the radio off its perch. It hit the floor with a loud thud and went dead. Everyone froze, staring at the eerily quiet box.

Mr. Marshall sighed, pinching the bridge of his nose. “Well, seems like we're *all* getting the silent treatment tonight, then.”

Blackout Shenanigans

It was 1942, and the blackout drills in London had become routine, but that didn’t make them any less chaotic. Mr. Albert Higgins had a plan, though; he liked to boast about his "preparedness" for the lights going out, and he was all set to prove it.

So he invited his neighbors over for tea: Mrs. Jenkins, the widow from across the street; Dr. Reginald Collins, the retired army doctor; and young Tommy, the street urchin who had taken to reading under the streetlamp outside. “No better time than a blackout for a good cup of tea," Albert said as he pulled out his "finest" teacups, which were the most mismatched set of mugs anyone could possibly have collected together.

As they settled in, the air-raid siren wailed, followed by the familiar click of the lights going out: the blackout had begun. Ready for action, Albert grabbed his flashlight—only to fumble and send it flying across the room. "Keep calm!" he declared in the dark.

Mrs. Jenkins let out a snort. "Don't worry, Albert. We won't dash just yet."

Tommy, more nimble than the rest, had already crawled across the floor and located the flashlight. He switched it on—just as it was pointed directly into Mrs. Jenkins' face. "Blimey!" she yelped, shielding her eyes.

Albert, moving toward the window to make sure his blackout curtains were properly drawn, jumped at the shrill cry. He tripped over the rug, careened into the table, and knocked over the teapot. Scalding liquid poured across the floor—and just where Reginald's foot happened to be.

"Ah! God save us all!" Reginald cried as he leaped out of his chair and into the darkness.

The siren wound down and the drill ended. The lights flickered back on to reveal utter chaos: Tommy prone on a soggy carpet, Reginald hopping beside his overturned chair, Mrs. Jenkins stumbling blindly, and Albert somehow wrapped in the blackout curtains like a ghost.

Albert sighed. “Well, I wasn't prepared for *this*.”

Sticky Tongue

It was a bone-chilling winter morning in 1948, and Frank Matthews was trudging through the snow to school with his best friend, Steve. The war was long over, but Frank still had battles he wanted to fight—especially against boredom. In this combative state of mind, he spotted the school door. The steel handle was shimmering with a layer of ice so thick it looked like a frosted cake.

“Bet you won’t lick it,” Steve smirked, throwing down the gauntlet.

Unfortunately, Frank could never refuse a dare. So he puffed out his chest. “Piece of cake.”

Now, every kid in the 1940s knew about the danger of frost and metal, but Frank was too eager to prove his mettle. He leaned in, stuck out his tongue, and *splat!* There was contact.

For a split second, nothing happened. Then, the horror quickly set in, along with the frost.

Frank's tongue was stuck solid. In a panic, he tried to yank his head back. But the door handle held firm like a steel trap.

Steve's face went pale. "Oh no, Frank! I think you're—"

"I kno'! I kno'!" Frank mumbled as his eyes darted around, hoping for a miracle. Other school kids gathered around, whispering and giggling at the spectacle. In no time at all, the morning bell rang.

Mrs. O'Malley, no-nonsense as ever, marched over. "What's all this fuss about?" Her thick eyebrows shot up when she saw Frank attached to the door like a human barnacle.

"Oh, for heaven's sake," she muttered. "This again?"

Frank's face was redder than his tongue as Mrs. O'Malley disappeared into the school. A moment later, she returned with a huff and a kettle of warm water, calmly pouring it over the frosty handle until Frank's tongue peeled away. He gasped like he'd been rescued from drowning.

"Frank," Mrs. O'Malley said, shaking her head. "You ought to pay attention to your schoolwork, young man."

Frank nodded mutely, while Steve grinned. "You really got into hot water there, mate!"

Stocking Stripes

It was 1944, and good nylons were simply impossible to come by. With rationing in full swing, women had to get creative if they wanted to look fashionable. Mary Thompson was no exception. Determined to keep up appearances for her night out at the dance hall, she decided to fake her nylons using the latest trend: drawing seams on the backs of her legs with eyebrow pencil. Easy peasy!

Standing in front of her mirror, Mary carefully bent down, dragging the pencil straight along her legs. “Look at that,” she said, admiring her handiwork. “No one will ever know.”

Her son Billy watched from the doorway, eyes wide with curiosity. “What are you doing, Mom?”

“Oh, just a little fashion trick, sweetie,” she said, shooing his ever-curious hand away. “Don’t touch! It needs to dry.”

Satisfied with her "stockings," Mary grabbed her purse and kissed her husband goodbye. “Don’t wait up,” she said with a coy smile.

At the dance hall, everything went splendidly. She swayed to the music, chatted with old friends, and felt every bit the glamorous woman she was. But halfway through the night, she felt a tap on her shoulder. It was Betty, her nosy neighbor. “Mary, dear,” she whispered, stifling a giggle, “you might want to check the back of your legs.”

Confused, Mary excused herself to the ladies' room and looked in the mirror. To her horror, the heat and humidity from the crowded dance hall had caused her "seams" to smudge. Instead of sleek, straight lines, she had squiggly marks running up her legs like a deranged train route.

“Oh no!” She tried to rub them off, which made things worse; it looked like Billy had made a mess on her legs with his crayons.

With a scoff, Mary returned to the dance floor, head held high as she spied Betty smirking at her. “I... I'm just setting a new trend!"

"What, abstract art stockings?" Betty chuckled.

Mary giggled despite herself. "You'll see, they'll be all the rage!"

Radio Days

In 1947, Saturday nights at our place meant gathering around the big wooden radio to listen to *The Adventures of Philip Marlowe*, a thrilling detective show. My sister Susie and I loved it so much that we wanted to put on our own version, mimicking the dramatic voices and mysterious plots we heard each week.

So, one evening, I jumped up. “Let’s do our own detective show! You be the damsel in distress, and I’ll be Detective Marlowe!” Susie eagerly agreed, and we set to work, gathering props: an old trench coat from Dad’s closet, a magnifying glass, and a broken broomstick for a walking cane.

Susie began by clutching her hand to her forehead dramatically. “Detective Marlowe! There’s been a terrible crime!”

Swimming in the trench coat, I growled, “Don’t worry, ma’am, I’ll solve the case.” I squinted through the magnifying glass at the family dog, Rusty, snoozing in the corner. “Hmm, this mutt is hiding something!”

I then poked Rusty with the broomstick, trying to get him to play along. But Rusty, startled, leaped up and knocked over a lamp. It fell to the floor with a loud crash, shards scattering everywhere.

“Uh-oh,” Susie whispered. “Mom’s gonna kill us!”

But I stayed in character. “Aha, the culprit has left clues!” I declared confidently as I grabbed a bottle of flour from the kitchen cupboard. “Let's dust them for fingerprints!” I tried to toss a bit of flour on the floor—only to accidentally empty half the bottle all over the kitchen and leave a fine white layer over everything, poor Rusty included!

Just then, my parents walked in. Mom's eyes widened at the mess—a broken lamp, a flour-coated dog, and two guilty kids caught red-handed (or rather, white-handed).

"What in the world—" Dad started, but then I raised my "cane" high.

"Fear not! I have solved the case!"

Mom deadpanned. "That's good, Mr. Detective, because I think that was your last case... *ever*."

Only then did I realize my parents were there. *Gulp.*

Bringing In the Ice

In 1941, the Wilsons had just gotten their brand-new icebox—a big, shiny refrigerator that needed to be manually stocked with ice. Young Charlie, always eager to show off his brawn, had been given the task of bringing in the ice block just dropped in by the delivery truck. He stood proud as his mom handed him a towel and pointed toward the massive chunk of ice sitting on the curb.

Charlie set off with determination. With gusto, he wrapped the towel around the ice, blew on his hands to warm them up, and tugged.

It didn't budge.

He grunted and tried again. The ice remained stubbornly glued to the spot like a statue.

From the front porch, his older sister Margaret smirked by the doorframe, arms crossed. “Need help there, Hercules?”

Charlie shot her a look. “I’ve got it!” He gave it one last heave, and the block shifted. It was barely an inch, but it was enough to knock him off balance. With a yelp, he lost his grip, and the ice slid out of the towel—and onto his foot.

“Ow!” He hopped on one foot while clutching the other. The ice took the opportunity to slide merrily down the sidewalk like a runaway train.

Margaret burst into laughter, clutching her sides. "'Ice' work, Charlie! You’re a real strongman now!”

Charlie limped down the sidewalk after the ice, nearly tripping over a milkman’s crate on the way. Finally, he stopped it by diving onto it like a football player recovering a fumble. They both slid to a stop just at the feet of one of their neighbors, who regarded Charlie like a judge at the Olympics about to give a failing score.

Breathless and red-faced, he dragged the ice back to the house and dumped it into the icebox with a loud thud, sweat dripping down his forehead.

“Top marks for finesse, Charlie,” Margaret teased.

Charlie glared at her as he closed the icebox door. "Cool it with the comments, would you?"

Ration Card Cuisine

It was 1943, and food rationing was in full swing. Mrs. Mildred Parker, the resourceful homemaker, had made it her personal mission to turn every meal into a gourmet experience, but her pantry was stocked with little more than flour, powdered eggs, and the dreaded cans of Spam. Her husband, George, wasn't exactly thrilled with the menu.

"Spam again?" George asked, peeking over her shoulder as she stood at the stove, stirring something that looked suspiciously like... well, like Spam.

"It's not just Spam," Mildred said, tapping the spoon on the pan with a grin. "Tonight, we're having *chicken*."

George raised an eyebrow. "Chicken? Are you sure? Because that looks like Spam. It smells like Spam..."

"Trust me," she said, winking. "By the time I'm done with it, you won't know the difference."

Mildred had found an article in *Housewives Weekly* titled "How to Make Spam Taste Like Chicken," and she was following it to the letter. After George left, she added the secret ingredient: chicken bouillon powder dissolved in water.

To complete the magic trick, she then coated the Spam mixture in flour, sprinkled it with salt and pepper, and fried it up like a real chicken cutlet.

George sat down at the table warily. Mildred placed the “chicken” in front of him with a flourish. “Voilà! Chicken à la Parker.”

He cut into the Spam and took a bite, chewing slowly and suspiciously. Mildred watched, her hands clasped together in anticipation.

“Well?” she asked.

George swallowed and stared at the ceiling. “It’s… it’s not terrible. Tastes like—”

“Chicken!” Mildred interrupted, her face lighting up.

“I was going to say rubber. But sure, chicken,” George muttered, taking another bite. “You know, if chickens were made of processed ham and salt.”

Mildred gave him a playful swat. “Oh, hush! Any more snark from you, and it will be powdered eggs for a week.”

George blanched, then smacked his lips together. “Well now, this *chicken* tastes utterly wonderful!”

The Radio Soap That Ruined a Life

It was 1946, and Mrs. Edith Perkins had a single great passion in life: her radio soap opera, *When A Girl Marries*. Every afternoon, she would settle into her favorite armchair and lose herself in the tumultuous lives of the characters. It was her escape from the ration books, her grumpy husband Harold, and the demands of post-war life.

"Edith, are you listening to me?" Harold grumbled from across the room one day, trying to get her attention by rattling his newspaper. Edith, however, was deep in the drama of star-crossed lovers Joan and Harry. Joan had just discovered a dark secret from Harry's past, and Edith was holding her breath.

"I knew it!" she gasped, clutching the armrest. "He's been lying to her this whole time!"

Harold blinked. "Who on Earth are you talking about?"

Edith shushed him like a child. "Not now, Harold! This is important!" Her eyes were glued to the radio as Joan wept into the sound of violins, sobbing, "How could you keep this from me, Harry?"

When the show ended on yet another cliffhanger, Edith was a wreck. "I can't believe him," she muttered to herself. "I knew Harry was trouble. I told Joan to be careful!"

Harold sighed. “You do know Joan's not real, right?”

Edith shot him a look. “She’s real to me! She’s been through so much, Harold. You just don’t understand.”

Harold nodded. "I certainly don't."

The next morning, Edith went to Mr. Hutch, the butcher, still stewing over the show's revelations. As she waited for her cut of meat, Mr. Hutch asked her how she was.

“Oh, not good,” she sighed. “Joan’s life is falling apart.”

Mr. Hutch frowned. “Joan?”

“Yes, Joan! The poor thing found out Harry's been lying to her all along! What will she do now?”

The butcher blinked, clearly confused. “Things will work out, I'm sure.”

Edith scoffed. “No, that's not all how these things go! Honestly, men...”

Mr. Hutch watched her storm away. "Was it something I said...?"

Ironing and Rags Gone Wrong

It was 1945, and Sally Holloway was determined to have perfectly straight hair for her date with her beau, Travis, who had recently returned from the war.

But with salons in short supply and no fancy hair straighteners, Sally had to get creative.

She'd heard from a friend that ironing her hair was the latest DIY trick. So, in her kitchen, Sally set up the ironing board and plugged in the iron. She'd tied some of her hair up in rags to create a few fashionable curls, leaving the rest of it to iron straight. Carefully, she laid a section of her hair on the board, holding her breath as she pressed the iron down.

"Ouch!" she yelped as she accidently singed a bit of her scalp.

Undeterred, she tried again with a towel between the iron and her hair. It worked! She straightened section after section, pleased with her work. But just as she finished ironing and began pulling out the rags from her hair, she heard a knock at the door.

"Travis!" she gasped.

Panicking, she rushed to smooth out her dress. With the front of her hair perfectly straight and elegant, she felt like a movie star. But in her haste, she forgot about the rags still hanging from the back of her head like forgotten party favors.

She opened the door, and there stood Travis, beaming and holding flowers.

He struggled to keep a straight face. "Sally, uh… Is that a new style?"

Sally blinked, confused, until she felt the weight of the rags dangling down her back. Mortified, she spun around and caught a glimpse of herself in the hallway mirror. There they were: rags and ringlets sticking out of her hair like errant clothes pegs.

Travis burst out laughing. “I think I like the little extra flair you've got going on!”

Sally groaned, yanking at her hair. “If you tell anyone about this, Travis, I swear…”

“Your secret’s safe with me, doll.” Travis chuckled, leaning in to kiss her cheek. "For now."

Sally groaned again.

Mom's Canning Factory

In 1943, our mom heard from her friends at church that preserving food was a great way to make supplies last longer, especially with all the rationing going on. So she transformed our small kitchen into what she proudly called the “Cooper Canning Factory.” Her first (and only) recruits were my sister Doris and me.

Mom started with tomatoes, lining up mason jars and lids for them. "This is teamwork!" she announced with gusto. "If we all do our part, we'll have food for winter!"

Tasked with washing tomatoes, I remember rolling my eyes in boredom. I dunked tomatoes in water and spun them around like a top, splashing water everywhere like a puppy being bathed. Doris was in charge of filling the jars, but she also furtively snacked on the tomatoes, eating more than she packed. That is until Mom gently rapped her shoulder with a frown.

As she chopped tomatoes, Mom misjudged the size of her pot and poured in too much water. The pot began to bubble and hiss, and steam filled the kitchen.

"Mom, it's a volcano!" I shrieked gleefully as the pot boiled over. Mom rushed to lift it off the stove but slipped, and a wave of tomato lava splashed onto the counter.

"Oh no!" Mom tried to mop up the mess with a dish towel while an oblivious Doris grabbed a lid, declaring, "I'm the jar inspector!" She clamped the lid down on one jar with too much force and not enough accuracy.

Just then, Dad walked in. He was greeted by a steamy, tomato-splattered kitchen, jars scattered everywhere, and the two of us laughing while Mom looked ready to collapse.

"Having fun, are we?" he grinned.

"Oh yes," Mom snarked, wiping tomato juice from her forehead. "Nothing like good old-fashioned canning!"

"Well, I hope you're ready for winter," Dad chuckled, glancing at the single, lopsided jar they'd managed to seal so far.

Mom sighed. "Winter? At this rate, I'll be lucky if we're ready for next week!"

Hollywood Glamour On A Budget

In 1947, sixteen-year-old Daisy Monroe had one goal in life: to look like a Hollywood starlet. Inspired by magazines full of glamorous photos of Ava Gardner and Rita Hayworth, Daisy decided she'd recreate the looks herself despite living on a modest budget in a small town. She convinced her friend Lila to join her on a trip to the local thrift store, where they'd be sure to find all the "essentials."

The first find was a dress that, in Daisy's words, "screamed red carpet." Lila thought it screamed something else entirely, but she kept that to herself. It was a massive purple gown with layers of taffeta that made Daisy look like an overgrown grape. But she persisted, gathering fistfuls of fabric at her waist. "We can just pin it here and here, and it'll be like the dresses in Vogue."

Next, Daisy spotted a faux fur stole that she thought rivaled anything Bette Davis wore. She tossed it around her shoulders with flair. “Very dramatic,” Lila said, trying to keep a straight face. Much later, they would realize the “fur” was shedding, leaving little clumps of fluff everywhere they went.

Finally, Daisy found a lopsided feathered hat that looked like it had once been a tortured flamingo. She pinned it to her curls and struck a pose. “Well, Lila?” she asked, hand on her hip. “Do I look like Ava?”

Lila tried not to laugh. “Oh, definitely. Maybe if Ava Gardner had a sister whom the family tried to hide in the attic.”

When Daisy proudly strutted down Main Street later that day, feeling like she was walking the red carpet, she did turn heads, though—mostly in confusion and some amusement at the trail of off-white clumps in her wake.

That evening, Daisy returned home with feathers askew, dress wrinkled, and fur barely there, but grinning ear to ear. “Who knew glamour could be this affordable?”

Her mother shook her head and sighed. "Who knew glamour could be so... unglamorous?"

Streetcar Shenanigans

In 1942, the bustling streetcars of Chicago were a marvel and a mystery to young Robbie Jenkins, newly fourteen. He'd heard all kinds of tales from his older brother, who claimed riding one was "like a rollercoaster, but for grown-ups." Determined to try one himself, Robbie bolted down to Main Street with a nickel to catch the next streetcar heading downtown.

As he climbed aboard, he was hit with a wave of excitement—and a gust of air that knocked his hat off. After fetching it from the ground, he tried to look cool, like the other passengers reading newspapers or quietly gazing outside. The conductor nodded at Robbie, and he grinned back, feeling like a "real" city person.

The streetcar jolted forward, and Robbie lurched, grabbing for a pole to steady himself. But he missed and landed on an elderly lady's lap, his hands ultimately grabbing something they probably shouldn't have. "Easy there, son," she kindly chuckled, noticing how nervous he was. Robbie's cheeks were bright red as he apologized.

As the streetcar filled up, it became easier to stay balanced with each stop and start. But when the car suddenly halted at Elm Street, Robbie wasn't prepared. He stumbled right into a businessman with a briefcase. The man glared at him and grumbled something about "young hooligans." Robbie mumbled sheepishly, pretending to study a map above the windows so he wouldn't make eye contact.

The ride continued, and Robbie spotted his stop coming up. He stepped up to the back door, but the streetcar jerked forward hard, causing him to stumble—and smack his face right into the glass. The other passengers stifled laughs as Robbie unsteadily leaped off the streetcar, cheeks flushed and stinging.

He looked back at the streetcar as it rumbled away, its passengers still looking amused. Robbie took a deep breath, brushed off his jacket, and straightened up.

"I should stick to walking," he muttered but managed a smile as he strode off—he couldn't help feeling a little more grown-up after all!

Rationing and Hand-Me-Downs

In 1944, with fabric rationed and clothes in short supply, Mom had come up with a creative (if slightly questionable) solution to clothe her three kids. She'd spent a weekend transforming the old, flower-printed curtains from our living room into "new" outfits. My six-year-old sister Annie thought it was wonderful to be wearing flowers, but my teenage self was mortified.

The day we first wore the new outfits to church was a memorable one. Annie happily twirled in her little floral dress as we walked in, oblivious to the giggles from other kids. She chirped, “Look, Mama, I’m a flower garden!”

Things were rather less delightful for me. My new shirt had once been the curtain valance, an especially loud pattern of bright, oversized roses. Every few steps, I tugged at it, feeling like a laundry line someone had hung bedlinen on.

During the service, I prayed harder than I’d ever prayed before that no one would recognize the shirt’s origins. But after the service, my hair stood on end as old Mrs. Hattie from down the street approached, squinting at me through her thick glasses.

“Oh my goodness, Kenny!” she cackled, pointing at my shirt. “Why, I believe I’ve seen those roses somewhere before!”

My face must have been as red as the aforementioned roses. “N-no, ma’am, I think you’re mistaken.”

“Honey, I’ve seen that curtain pattern every time I came over for bridge!" Mrs. Hattie winked. "Your mother’s got a fine eye for recycling.”

I wanted to sink through the floorboards. But then Annie piped up, “Mama says we’re fashion pioneers!”

Just then, another churchgoer passed by, whispering to her friend, "You know, that's not a bad idea. I have some old curtains that would make for a lovely skirt!"

So, as we left the church, Mom smiled proudly and patted me on the back while I groaned. "See, son? You're setting a trend!"

I sighed. "It's going to be the tablecloth next, isn't it?"

The Day the Horse Decided Not to Go to School

In 1941, we Peterson kids had our own "school bus": the family horse, Buttercup. Buttercup was usually a sweet, reliable mare—but one blustery autumn morning, she woke up in a mood.

Elsie, the oldest, clambered onto Buttercup's back, with my older brother Sam and I perched behind her. With lunch pails swinging, we set off down the dirt road. But only a few minutes in, Buttercup came to a complete stop right in the middle of the road. Elsie nudged her gently. "Come on, Buttercup, we're gonna be late!"

Buttercup flicked her tail, unimpressed.

Sam gave her a little kick. "Let's go, girl!" Buttercup let out a snort that sounded like a laugh.

I giggled. “She says no!”

Undeterred, Elsie whispered sweetly in Buttercup’s ear, like she’d seen Pa do. “Please, Buttercup? School’s just down the road.”

Buttercup munched on a patch of grass beside the road, utterly indifferent to our plight.

We were frantic. Other children walking by on foot laughed as they passed. “Gonna set up camp there?” a neighbor boy jeered.

Sam tried a different tactic. “If you get us to school, Buttercup, I’ll give you an extra apple!” Buttercup’s ears perked up—she started to plod forward.

But just as we reached the final stretch, Buttercup spotted a familiar field she liked to graze in. With a sudden gleam in her eye, she made a sharp turn, ignoring all our protests, and trotted straight into the field, where she dropped down to roll in the grass.

We three tumbled off, lunch pails flying, landing in a heap. Covered in dust and bits of grass, we watched as Buttercup stood up, looking pleased with herself, and happily munched some spilled apples from our lunch pails.

The teacher standing at the school entrance looked severe at first, but her expression softened when she saw the hay in our hair and the look of defeat in our eyes. "Your mare had her way with you, did she? Come on in then, quickly now!"

The 1950s

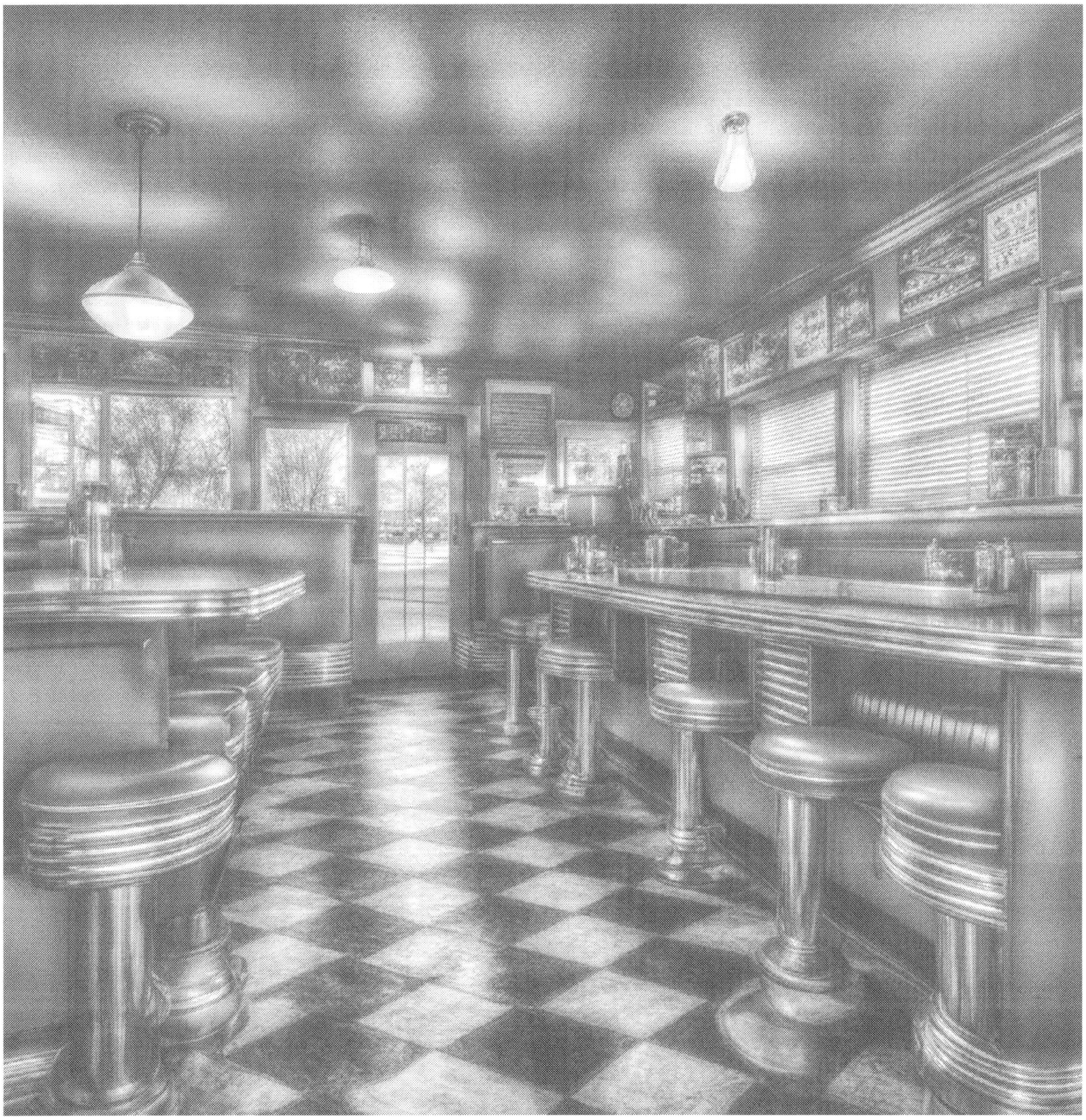

When Snowy Static Was High-Tech

In 1955, my family got our first television set: a chunky box with a tiny screen and more wood paneling than our kitchen. It was the marvel in the middle of the living room; the picture was the closest thing to magic I'd ever seen—when it actually appeared. Most of the time, though, all we got was static, which Dad called "high-tech snow."

The antenna was the star of our daily comedy show. Every evening, we'd gather around the set, and Dad would issue orders like a military general. He'd twist the antenna left and right or hold it in various directions, squinting at the screen whenever he could see it. Mom, who wasn't tech savvy, would hold her breath while my little sister Kathy and I crouched like soldiers, awaiting Dad's instructions.

One night, Dad enlisted Uncle Charlie into our campaign. Charlie was taller than Dad, very skinny, and could fall over in a strong enough wind, but he'd do anything for a slice of Mom's homemade pie.

So we had Uncle Charlie stand on a chair with the antenna held high in his hands while we shouted instructions like "A little left!" or "Tilt it away from us!" And, miracle of miracles, we got the picture! The only problem? Charlie had to stand perfectly still on his chair, or the static would return.

"I think I'm cramping up," I heard him mutter, but Dad hushed him.

For nearly an hour, Uncle Charlie stayed there like a statue. We got through half of *I Love Lucy* before his legs finally gave way—and he fell off the chair with a crash! Luckily, the only things that broke were the antenna and Charlie's dignity, and Mom's pie helped compensate for the latter problem.

While Dad eventually found a way to mount the antenna on our ceiling and get a steadier reception, I don't think anything on television was ever as exciting as that evening with Uncle Charlie!

Ironing Out the Wrinkles

In 1958, Louise Madsen's ironing ritual was a performance art piece. Every Tuesday morning, she'd waltz into the kitchen, fling open the fridge, and start pulling out stacks of cotton shirts, pillowcases, and even the odd pair of her husband John's boxers. The whole pile, cool as cucumbers, was stored in the fridge like leftovers.

One day, her young grandson Ben watched this strange, frosty laundry parade and just had to ask: “Grandma, why do you keep clothes in the fridge?”

She gave Ben a look like he'd just asked why the sky was blue.

“If you dampen them and put them in the fridge, they're easier to iron,” she said. “See, you don't have to re-wet them every time you move the iron.”

Ben nodded along like someone who was only pretending to understand; Louise laid a cold shirt on the ironing board and started smoothing it out with her heavy iron. As she worked, Ben couldn't help but notice an entirely different set of wrinkles: the fine lines on her arms.

Trying to be clever, he winked, "Hey, Grandma, can you iron the wrinkles out of your arm, too?"

Louise stopped mid-press, looked at Ben over her glasses, and let out a laugh so loud it nearly sent the clothes stack flying across the room. "Ha! If only it were that easy. But let me tell you a secret," she said, putting the iron aside. "Wrinkles are a sign of character and happiness. That's why people like me with wrinkles a-plenty are such rich and lively folk. Isn't that right, John?"

John, who had just walked in, looked utterly confused. Louise nudged him for an answer, so he provided one: "Yes, young Ben, your Grandma is certainly a character, that's for sure! Can't iron that out in a hurry!"

Louise responded by indignantly smacking John in the arm with his freezing boxers, and Ben couldn't help chuckling as his Grandpa yelped at the frosty touch.

The King and the Swoon

It was 1956, and the biggest thing to hit Olivia Glendale's town wasn't the new supermarket or even the milkshake machine at Bob's Diner—it was Elvis Presley on TV. She had heard the rumors and whispers from the girls at school about his hair, his voice, his *hips*. But it wasn't enough to prepare her for the night she first beheld his glory.

Olivia's family were crammed into the living room, the TV humming and glowing like a spaceship. Mr. Glendale was grumbling about "these new-fangled rock 'n' rollers" while Mrs. Glendale waved him off, secretly more excited than she'd admit. As soon as Elvis came on screen, the air practically buzzed. His voice was butter, his hair was slick, and when he moved, Olivia's heart did a little dance that made her feel dizzy.

She was leaning forward, practically glued to the screen, when Elvis shot a smile at the camera—*the* smile. Suddenly, Olivia's legs went weak, and the next thing she knew, she was swaying, tilting, and then... *Bam*! She hit the wall with the grace of a toppling ironing board.

Mr. Glendale snapped up from his armchair. "What in the—?" Mrs. Glendale rushed over to check on her suddenly faintish daughter.

Olivia's face was redder than a ripe tomato, but she managed to squeak, "I... I just tripped."

Mr. Glendale looked suspicious. “Tripped? Or swooned?”

“Dad! Girls like me don’t—” Olivia began to insist. But then Elvis did one of his iconic hip shakes, and her legs betrayed her again, sending her stumbling into Mrs. Glendale's arms.

“Looks like Elvis here gave you a case of the swoons!” Mrs. Glendale giggled as she patted her arm.

For days after, Olivia's parents teased her relentlessly. Mr. Glendale started calling Elvis the “heartthrob hooligan” and even tried (and failed) to mimic his moves—much to Mrs. Glendale’s horror. When Elvis next appeared on the screen, Olivia made sure to sit down and firmly grip her chair, which had a label on it as a reminder: "The Swoon Seat."

Poodle Skirts

I got my most infamous nickname at the Spring Sock Hop of 1957, and it all began with my swanky outfit. My mom and I spent weeks picking out fabric, stitching, and sewing, and in the end, my poodle skirt was a masterpiece: bright red with a little black poodle, rhinestone collar, and a leash that looped around my waist. I looked like I’d strutted right off a magazine cover!

When we walked into the school gym, heads turned. I was floating on air, twirling and showing off my skirt to anyone who would look. I even spotted

Jimmy Baxter, the cutest boy in school, giving me the once-over. He flashed a grin, and my heart did a little flip. I was so busy staring back that I didn't notice the decorations hanging just a little too low above the punch bowl.

Suddenly, as I leaned in for some punch, I felt warmth by my hip—and not the kind Jimmy Baxter gave me. I looked down in horror—the edge of my poodle skirt had brushed the flame of a candle on the table and was smoldering! Panic set in, and I started flapping my skirt, trying to blow it out, which only fanned the flames higher.

Within seconds, my friend Peggy was screaming, "Rachel's on fire!" Teachers and students alike whipped around as I tried to stay calm—although I mostly just spun in circles, which didn't help.

Mr. Delaney, the gym teacher, raced over with his jacket, ready to tackle me to the floor. But before he could, Peggy dumped an entire ladle of punch on me! Jimmy then heroically tossed his cup of root beer in for good measure.

I stood there, blushing and soaked in punch and soda, with the charred edge of my poodle skirt smelling like a burnt marshmallow. Jimmy gave me an awkward thumbs-up, and I laughed because my brain couldn't think of anything better to do instead.

And that's how I came to be known as "Red Hot Rachel."

Accidental Soda Jerk

In 1959, Mel's Diner needed a replacement soda jerk for a day. It was the hottest spot in town, where all the cool kids hung out, so Mel's nephew Dalton was thrilled at being chosen for the job—even if it was only because he happened to be at the diner by accident.

Mel handed Dalton the soda fountain like he was giving him the keys to a Cadillac. "Don't mess up." Dalton nodded as confidently as he could, looking like a reed wobbling in the breeze.

The first order was simple: one chocolate malt, extra thick. Dalton fumbled around, pouring chocolate syrup and milk, and threw in a little more chocolate for the extra thickness. But when he turned on the mixer, he forgot to put the lid on, and a chocolate explosion painted the walls—and Dalton.

Then came the double strawberry shakes for Patty and her friends, who were regulars with very high standards. Dalton made those shakes like his life depended on it, only to realize he'd used vanilla syrup instead of strawberry. He put in red coloring and served them anyway, hoping they wouldn't notice, but within seconds, Patty shrieked, "This isn't strawberry!" Mel shot Dalton a glare that could curdle milkshakes.

At that point, a couple of boys from the football team started teasing Patty, saying she couldn't handle a little vanilla. Patty fired back that their chocolate shake looked more like muddy water; milkshake insults soon flew across the diner like spitballs. Someone flung a spoonful of whipped cream, which hit Patty right on the nose, and then the whole place erupted in a full-on milkshake war.

Strawberry, chocolate, vanilla—it was chaos! Mel was hollering, “I’m not paying for this mess!” as whipped cream dripped from the ceiling. By the end, the diner looked like a tornado had chucked a dairy farm at it.

Dalton couldn't be discharged from duty quickly enough. But his legend lived on as "The Jerk" who started the Great Milkshake War of ’59.

The Jelly Menu

In 1954, Wilma Woodrow decided that Thanksgiving needed a little “modern flair.” The woman had discovered gelatin molds and was convinced that everything tasted better in wobbly, colorful jelly. So, she came up with the brilliant (and terrifying!) idea of a menu where *every single dish* was suspended in gelatin.

When her children and grandchildren arrived at her house, the dining table looked like a science experiment gone wrong. The centerpiece was a lime green turkey, complete with little pimentos for eyes and a celery stick for a beak. It jiggled ominously every time someone walked by; her eldest, Lou, swore he saw it blink!

"Oh, isn't it festive?" Wilma beamed as she set out even more "delicacies": cranberry jelly shaped like a flower pot, stuffing in an amber-colored gelatin, and a neon-orange carrot and raisin "salad" that looked more like a lava lamp than food.

Her daughter Judy looked pitiable as she reached for the mashed potato jelly mold, topped with a perfect gelatin gravy pool in the middle. She poked at it, and it wobbled so threateningly that she nearly shoved it down the table.

"Doesn't anyone want the green bean casserole?" Wilma asked, holding up a turquoise gelatin mold studded with floating green beans and crispy onions, like flies in sickly amber. The table went silent as everyone secretly weighed just how much Grandma's feelings were worth.

Then her youngest grandchild Mike piped up, "Is there any regular food?" Grandma dramatically clutched her apron.

"Why, of course, Mikey!" As she shuffled into the kitchen, everyone very quickly passed their plates to Lou—who discreetly tossed their dinner into the bush outside the window. Their plates looked quite neat when Wilma returned with dessert: a huge gelatin parfait tower in layers of orange, grape, and strawberry. Because, of course, it was!

In the end, Wilma's family may not have been entirely satisfied with the dinner, but the jiggly rainbow-colored memory of it was etched in their minds forever.

Wringer Washers Eat Things

In 1957, the Bellamy family still relied on an old wringer washer to tackle the laundry. Laura Bellamy was a whiz with it, but every time her daughter Irma tried to help, the machine developed a mind of its own.

One Saturday, Irma thought she'd surprise her mom by getting a jump on the laundry. She loaded the washer, set the agitator whirling, and waited for the fun part: feeding clothes through the wringer. She had her favorite T-shirt at the ready, and pushed it through with determination. But somehow, the machine grumbled and sucked it in like it was chewing bubble gum! In seconds, the shirt was twisted into a tight, damp spiral on the other side, and when Irma tried to pull it free, the wringer took that as an invitation to grab her hand.

The thing clamped down, and Irma yelped; she tried to pull her fingers free, but the wringer just kept chugging along, dragging her arm inch by inch. In a panic, she reached out with her other hand to hit the release button—and that hand got caught, too! There Irma was, elbows to the washer, wrestling with the thing like it was a wild animal.

Just then, her little brother Cody wandered in with a popsicle in hand. He took one look at Irma, trapped in the maw of the wringer, and burst out laughing. “You look like Mom’s pot roast!” he giggled.

“Get. Mom,” Irma managed to say through gritted teeth. Cody scurried off, still giggling, while Irma prayed arms wouldn’t end up as laundry spaghetti.

Laura finally burst through the door, and her face went from horror to laughter in seconds. She unplugged the machine and freed Irma's arms, which were red and wrinkled like prunes.

For weeks after, Cody told everyone how his sister was "gobbled up" by the washer. Irma was banned from laundry duty, but as far as she was concerned, it was the best ban she'd ever gotten by far!

Drag Races and Groundings

In 1958, Greg got it into his head that he was the coolest guy in town. His dad had just bought a new Plymouth sedan—a tank of a car with fins sharp enough to cut the air. Greg, however, was convinced it could beat anything on wheels. He bragged at school that he’d take anyone on in a race. His friends laughed, but Greg was determined to prove that the Plymouth wasn’t just some old car.

So one Friday night, he waited until his parents had fallen asleep, then snuck out, lifted his dad’s keys, and rolled the car down the driveway. The Plymouth was a behemoth that creaked like a rocking chair, but to Greg, it felt like a rocket ship.

When he reached the old road where his friends were waiting, Johnny, the local hot rod kid, was already there in his souped-up Chevy. Greg tried to play it cool, leaning against the Plymouth like James Dean. But Johnny just laughed. “You think that boat can take me?”

Greg puffed up. “Just watch.” So they lined up, and Greg’s heart pounded as they took off.

Well, *Johnny* took off, at least.

The Plymouth, on the other hand, roared for about two seconds, then choked, jerked, and settled into a pace that would be impressive—if he were delivering milk.

Greg tried everything: gripping the wheel tighter, yelling at the engine, even bouncing in the seat like that would somehow urge the car forward. Nothing worked. The Plymouth chugged along at its own leisurely pace, and when Greg made it to the finish line, Johnny had been waiting there long enough to polish his car twice if he wanted to.

To add insult to injury, Greg's dad was waiting on the porch when he finally got back home; Greg’s racing career was over before it started. He spent the next month grounded, washing the "rocket ship" every weekend—if only it could actually whisk him up and away to outer space!

Sneaking Into the Drive-in

In 1956, Leroy had one goal for the summer: sneak into the drive-in without paying a dime. He'd heard his older brother brag about "riding in the trunk" to save money, so Leroy was convinced he could pull it off, too. One night, he rounded up his buddies Bobby and Joe and convinced them that sneaking in would make them legends.

Bobby's cousin had an old Ford, so they came up with a flawless plan: Leroy would hide in the trunk with Joe while Bobby and his cousin paid for two tickets upfront. They waited until the ticket booth was in sight before cramming Leroy and Joe into the trunk, giving them a flashlight, and telling them to stay quiet. Leroy gave a thumbs-up, feeling like a real rebel.

As the car inched forward in line, things got hot—literally! Leroy started sweating buckets, feeling like he was in an oven. The car hit a bump, and he cracked his head against the trunk lid. He could smell wet socks, motor oil, and Joe's armpits, and he was starting to regret the plan.

Finally, he felt the car stop. But instead of driving into the lot, Bobby chatted for too long with the ticket lady. Curious, she asked them to pop the trunk for a “routine check,” and Bobby and his cousin panicked, not knowing what to say.

Leroy, unaware of the situation outside—and very aware of being pressed against Joe inside—thought it was his cue to get out. As the trunk popped open, he leaped out like a jack-in-the-box, only to come face-to-face with the startled ticket lady. She shrieked, he shrieked, and everyone else in line laughed while honking and pointing.

The ticket lady gave Leroy a lecture and made them buy extra tickets for him and Joe. And to top it off, Leroy watched the entire movie smelling like trunk grease and sweaty defeat. Leroy and Joe did become legends, though—the infamous "Trunk Lunks" of the drive-in!

Banned Brylcreem

In 1954, my cousin Danny was the coolest kid in town—or so he thought. His secret weapon? Brylcreem. Every morning, he’d slather his hair with that greasy, gooey stuff until it shone brighter than a Cadillac bumper. “Just a little dab,” he’d say, but his “dab” was practically half a bottle!

One Saturday, Danny came over to our house for dinner. He walked in, hair slicked back like an oil puddle and sat on Mom’s prized floral couch. She’d saved for months for that couch, and Danny plopped down without a thought, leaving an oily silhouette on the fabric. I could see Mom's eye twitching, but she somehow kept her cool.

When he leaned against the walls, he left greasy headprints; every chair he sat on had a stain where his head had rested on it. By the time he left, our house looked like it had been attacked by an army of oily ghosts. Mom spent the next hour scrubbing everything, muttering very impolite things about "that greasy menace."

Danny's hair obsession soon got him in real trouble. He was talking to Mary Lou, his latest crush, when his hair touched her shoulder. She gasped as a massive Brylcreem stain materialized on her sweater. Wrinkling her nose, she said, "Danny, you smell like a gas station!" and left him standing there, shining with embarrassment.

Mom had had enough, too. After Danny left a greasy spot on the backseat of Dad's brand-new car another time, she stormed over to Danny's house, knocked firmly on the door, and informed Aunt Rita that "Danny and his Brylcreem are officially banned from our household!" After that, Aunt Rita put him on a strict budget—one dab, a proper little one, and that was it.

Danny was crushed. He tried water, he tried combing his hair, but nothing gave him that signature shine. Without the gallons of grease, his hair went flat, and his expression followed suit. We didn't feel too bad for him, though!

Pin Curls and Cold Cream

In 1956, Violet's grandmother Ellen was a walking makeup tutorial. Every evening, she'd lock herself in the bathroom for hours, emerging with pin curls tight enough to bounce quarters off and a face slathered in cold cream so thick she looked like a ghost. She was sure it was the secret to keeping her youthful glow.

Violet, who dreamt of being a Hollywood star, watched Ellen's routine like it was the holy grail of beauty secrets. One evening, after Ellen went out for her weekly bridge game, Violet seized the opportunity. "If I'm going to be a glamour queen, it starts tonight."

Violet snuck into Ellen's bathroom and went straight for the cold cream. She scooped a glob out of the jar and slapped it on her face, practically slathering it up to her eyebrows until her face looked like she was auditioning for a horror movie. Then came the pin curls: Violet started rolling her hair in little twists and pinning them all over her head. The pins kept flopping, though, so she had to settle for a couple of half-twisted clumps, hoping it'd still look glamorous.

Feeling like a movie star, Violet struck poses in the mirror. She practiced her "sultry" face, pouting her lips and narrowing her eyes, going for a mysterious look that mostly resembled a bad squint. She was so absorbed in her "Hollywood transformation" that she didn't hear Ellen come home.

The bathroom door flew open, and there she stood, eyes wide, clutching her bridge purse. For a moment, she just stared. Then she burst out laughing so hard that she had to lean against the doorframe.

"What are you doing?" she managed, wiping tears from her eyes.

"Trying to be glamorous, Grandma!" Violet huffed, but it was hard to look too offended with cold cream dripping down her chin and pin curls dangling at odd angles.

"If that's what you're going for, honey," Grandma chuckled, "then you've got a long way to go!"

Ducktail Fails

In 1957, the only thing I wanted in life was a ducktail haircut that would make me look like James Dean. Every cool guy on TV had that slicked-back, perfectly swooping hairstyle, and I knew it would make me the talk of the town.

So I went to Joe's Barber Shop with a clear mission: "I want a ducktail." Joe raised an eyebrow but nodded, combing and clipping with the focus of a brain surgeon.

When he spun me around to face the mirror, I was horrified! The back of my head looked less like a duck's tail and more like a dead bird was half-buried in my hair: an uneven, lopsided wave that barely had a swoop. Determined to salvage my look, I paid him and told myself I could fix it at home.

I practically ran to my bathroom and grabbed Dad's old tube of Brylcreem, slathering on way more than any sane person would. But the more I added, the more my hair just... drooped. My "ducktail" looked like a greasy pancake, but I didn't give up. I borrowed my mom's hair dryer, hoping a little heat would "set the style"—which was definitely not how these things worked.

Just as I was blow-drying my dripping mop, the bathroom door opened, and my little sister barged in. She took one look at me, then started laughing so hard she was gasping for air. "You look like a porcupine!"

Then Mom walked in. She covered her mouth, clearly trying not to laugh, and said, "Do you really need all that grease, dear?"

Defeated, I washed my hair about six times before giving up. All the Brylcreem left it limp and lifeless, a tragic shadow of James Dean's iconic look. At school the next Monday, my friends took one look at my failed ducktail and dubbed me "Duck Disaster."

My hair eventually recovered, but the rest of me did not. This was a tale I would never go through again!

Tea Party for a Coronation

In 1953, Grandma Peggy decided to throw a tea party to celebrate Queen Elizabeth’s coronation. But this wasn’t just any tea party: Peggy insisted it be a masquerade tea party. "If we’re going to celebrate the Queen, we’re doing it right!" she declared, rummaging through her attic for anything even remotely British-looking.

On the big day, her living room was transformed into a makeshift throne room. Peggy had dug out lace doilies, her finest teapot, and a huge Union Jack that she’d taped to the wall. Her son Ralph showed up in a thrifted suit with a tin-foil crown, claiming to be “King Ralph of Liverpool.” Her daughter Betty wore her wedding dress, repurposing it as “British royalty chic” with a bunch of pearls that jingled every time she moved. And her grandson Brian was forced to be the “Royal Jester,” complete with a pointy hat Peggy made out of construction paper.

But it was Peggy who stole the show. She wore a dusty, bejeweled dress she swore was her grandmother’s Victorian ball gown, though it suspiciously resembled a tablecloth. She topped it off with a plastic tiara from Woolworths and a feather boa. “You may only address me as Your Majesty the Queen Mother,” she announced in an exaggerated British accent thicker than jam.

The tea itself was a comedy of errors. Grandma served cucumber sandwiches, but she used pickles instead of cucumbers. The look on Ralph's face after his first bite was priceless. The "scones," biscuits from a can, were so hard that Aunt Betty chipped a tooth trying to take a bite.

The tea was a mix of lemonade and iced tea, which was apparently "how the royals have it." But when she took a sip, she spat it back out again for how overly sweet it was! Everyone else was laughing so hard that she finally gave in, even graciously dropping her Queen Mother act in the process. "You'd think they'd know how to make decent tea over there by now!"

Where's the Party in a Party Line

In the 1950s, the Masons were one of the lucky families with a phone at home. The downside? They had to share a party line with half the neighborhood. Mrs. Mason called it progress, but Mr. Mason felt like he was living in a soap opera—and not one of the good ones either!

Anytime they picked up the phone, there was a good chance Mrs. Jenkins, the chatty neighbor, was telling her sister every tiny detail of her cat's latest misadventure. Sometimes, they'd overhear Mr. Sampson's long-winded debates with the hardware store on who'd ordered the wrong kind of nails. But there were good sides: young Ethan sometimes heard girls talking about him and the other boys in class in loud whispers and giggles.

One day, Mr. Mason was expecting an important business call, so he stationed himself near the phone. Just as it rang, he leaped to grab it, but Mrs. Jenkins was already mid-sentence about her new curtains.

“Mrs. Jenkins,” Mr. Mason said as politely as possible, “I have an urgent call coming. Mind hanging up?”

“Oh, of course, of course!” she replied—and stayed on for at least another minute, finishing up her curtain critique. Mr. Mason got his call, but the line was soon hijacked again. “Hello? Hello? Can y’all keep it down?” It was Mr. Sampson, complaining about hardware again. Soon after, one of the neighborhood teenagers chimed in, “Mr. Mason, we’re tryin’ to talk here!”

The call soon turned into utter chaos, with constant interruptions as three different groups of people tried to have their own conversations on the same line. Mr. Mason finally gave up, apologized to his business associate with a sigh, and hung up the phone, muttering darkly to himself.

"That's the price of progress, dear," Mrs. Mason said kindly. "Think of it as... oh, as a party!"

"A party? Ha!" Mr. Mason grumbled. "I've been to funeral parties that were more fun than this noise. Mark my words; all this gossiping and sharing lines together will never take off!"

The Great Jukebox Jam

It was 1957, and every Friday night, my friends and I would hit up Sal's Diner for milkshakes and tunes from the brand-new jukebox. Sal had just stocked it with the latest Elvis records, and that diner hadn't been the same since. But one day, there was a "little less conversation," a "little more action," and a little too much Elvis!

I'd just dropped in a nickel for "Hound Dog"; Elvis's voice filled the room, crooning about how we "ain't nothin' but a hound dog" as we spun and twirled like we were at the biggest sock hop in town. When the song ended, we were all breathless and ready to sit down, but suddenly, Elvis started up again. We just laughed, assuming someone else had picked the same song.

But then it happened again. And again. After the fifth round of "Hound Dog," Sal ran over to the jukebox, whacking it on the side like he could knock some sense into it. He poked buttons and hit switches, but Elvis just kept on telling us we "ain't nothin' but a hound dog."

By round seven, everyone was getting a little twitchy. Even Judy, whose locker was covered in Elvis pictures, was rolling her eyes. Sal gave the jukebox another mighty whack, but Elvis was going nowhere. People started to trickle out, holding their ears like they'd heard enough "Hound Dog" to last a lifetime.

When Mr. Thompson, our high school principal, walked in to grab a late-night coffee, he looked around in confusion as Elvis kept singing over and over.

“Sal,” he raised an eyebrow, “Sounds like you've got a bad case of Elvis fever.”

Finally, Sal got desperate. He pulled the jukebox’s plug, and with a dramatic pop, silence filled the diner. Then we all cheered like we’d just been liberated from prison.

Sal took the Jukebox Jam incident in good humor, though; a few days later, his diner had a new special hotdog offer on the menu—Hound Dogs!

The Phone Booth Challenge

In 1958, Eddie Weezer came up with “the challenge”—how many teenagers could fit into a single phone booth? The record at the time was something like fourteen, but Eddie was convinced his gang could beat it. “We’ve got practice squeezing into cars,” he boasted. “This’ll be a cinch!”

So one Saturday afternoon, they all piled into the parking lot outside Miller’s Drugstore, where the town’s one and only phone booth sat, glistening in the sunlight like a glass and metal trophy. Eddie was ready to be the first one in. He squeezed himself into the booth and crouched down, looking far too serious about it. “Next!” he yelled, waving like he was a carnival barker.

Calvin went in next, elbowing his way to a corner and curling up like a human pretzel. Then came Judy, who somehow managed to slide in and plop right on top of Calvin's foot. Soon, Bobby and Sue climbed in, followed by the Henderson twins, who somehow folded themselves like origami to fit along the back. The discomfort was piling on, but the taste of glory was still too tempting.

By the time nine people had squeezed into the booth, things were already getting weird. Bobby’s elbow was jammed into Eddie's side, and someone’s shoe was dangerously close to his face. Still, he called for more. “We’re gonna beat fourteen!” he declared.

With some more wiggling, they made it to twelve. Just when Calvin thought they couldn’t possibly fit anyone else, Gary—the biggest of the bunch—forced himself in and against the glass, squashing the rest against each other, and shut the door behind him. Thirteen teenagers in a phone booth!

But just then, a gust of wind rattled the door, and it flew open; Gary and the rest burst out like clowns from a clown car. Mrs. Patterson, the local librarian, happened to be walking by and stared at the heap of limbs that was Eddie's gang.

He simply shook his head. "Kids these days."

The 1960s

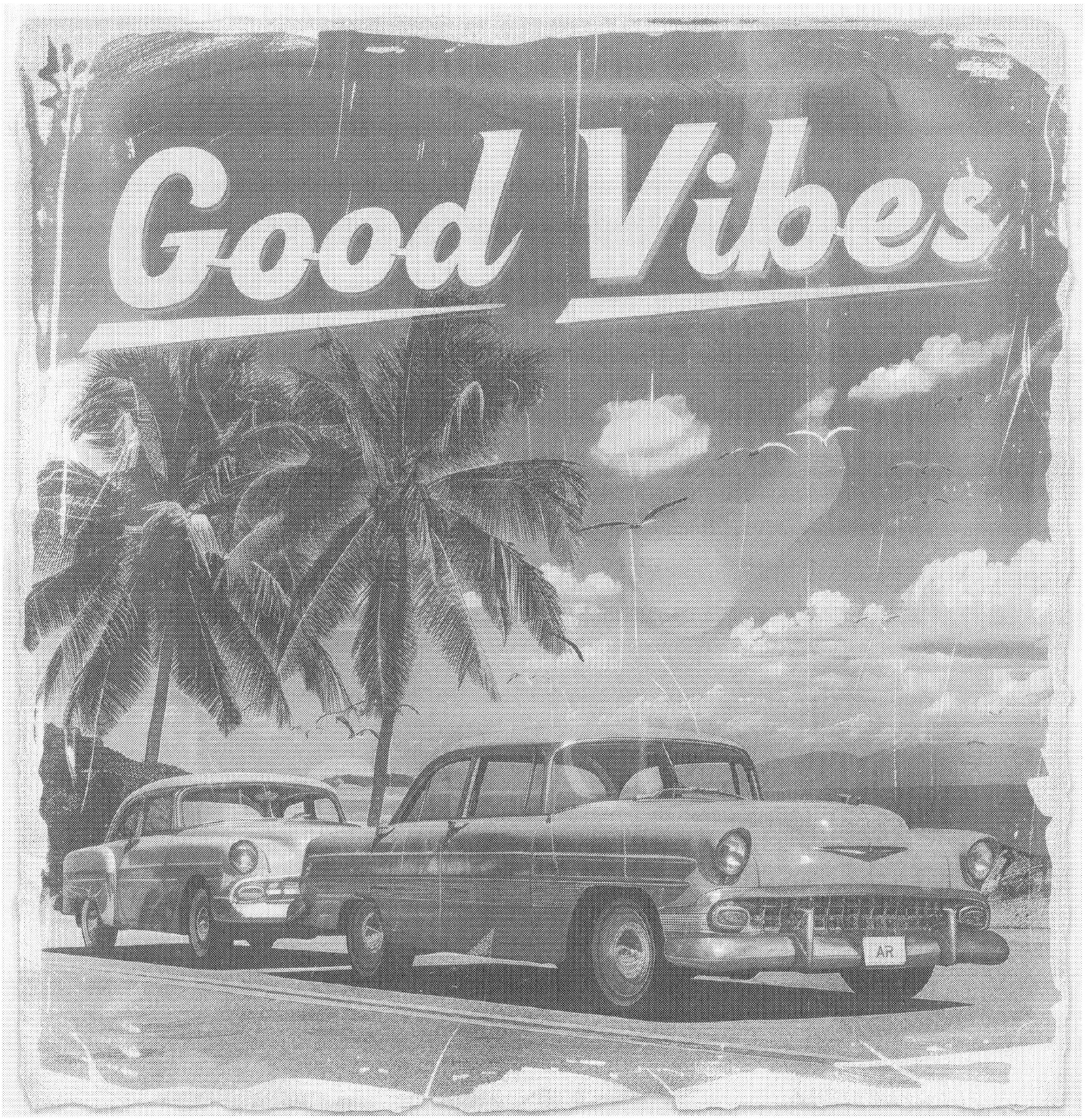

The Ultimate Beehive

In 1965, it was all about having the biggest, tallest, and most perfectly teased beehive hairdo in town. Sally Carmichael, the ultimate "it" girl, had her hair stacked so high she grazed low-hanging branches as she walked. But Nancy Weaver was determined to steal Sally's crown—both metaphorically and literally!

Nancy saved up for weeks to buy the biggest bottle of Aqua Net she could find, and after hours of careful teasing and twisting—and choking on hairspray fumes—she had herself a beehive that seemed to scrape the heavens. With her hair bobbing dangerously, she strutted into Mrs. Plum's dance hall on Friday night, winking at the boys and twirling proudly.

But Sally had noticed. With the unspoken challenge accepted, Sally snuck out to the powder room and started stacking her hive even higher. By the end of the night, people stopped noticing the girls below their monstrous beehives.

Not to be outdone, Nancy quickly stuffed her hive with anything she could find in her purse—tissues, gum wrappers, even a few pencils—to give it extra lift. For a grand finish, she grabbed a paper straw, fixed it to the top, and blew through it like a balloon, inflating her beehive a final inch.

The crowd went wild as Nancy wobbled forward with her masterpiece, bobbing and swaying under its weight. But just as she basked in victory, the unthinkable happened: a small gust from the open window.

One misplaced hairpin. A soft, horrifying *pop*.

With a dramatic poof, the entire thing collapsed in a cloud of Aqua Net and bobby pins. But just as Sally smirked from the sidelines, her own beehive lost a vital hairpin to the draft and came tumbling down around her.

Everyone roared with laughter as the two girls were left staring at their beehives in shambles on the floor. Then Sally and Nancy smiled wryly at each other, feeling like competing boxers at the end of a long fifteen rounds. It *had* been a good fight while it lasted, after all!

Moon Landing Malfunctions

It was July 20, 1969, and the Miller family was crowded around their living room TV, breathlessly waiting to watch Neil Armstrong make history by setting foot on the moon. Mr. Miller, a proud owner of the latest color TV—not that it mattered for a moon landing that would be in black-and-white—had invited half the neighborhood over to watch. The living room was packed, the air smelled of popcorn, and everyone was buzzing with excitement.

As Armstrong's foot hovered above the lunar surface, Mr. Miller dramatically shushed everyone. The anticipation was thick. Mrs. Pollock from next door clutched her pearls. But just as Armstrong opened his mouth to say those famous words, the TV screen flickered, buzzed, and then... static.

Everyone froze.

“No, no, no!” Mr. Miller leaped up, fiddling with the receiver. “Kelly, run up to the roof and check the antenna!”

Ten-year-old Kelly sprinted up the stairs while Mr. Miller frantically turned the dial. The crowd started murmuring, Mrs. Pollock switched to clutching her husband from her pearls, and old Mr. Dawkins muttered something about “dang newfangled technology.”

Kelly yelled down, “It looks fine, Dad!”

“Well, it’s not fine! Do something!” Mr. Miller shouted back. Just then, he had an idea. With everyone watching in tense silence, he gave the TV a firm whack. The static flickered, then cleared, revealing... Armstrong back on the lunar lander, and his “small step” had already been taken.

They had missed history.

“Nooooo!” Mrs. Pollock wailed, sinking to the floor. Mr. Miller stared at the TV in horror, then back at his guests in a mix of apology and frustration.

Frank from down the street tried to break the tension. “Well, we saw him just before he stepped down, right?” he chuckled. “I mean, it shouldn't be too hard to imagine how it looked!”

But nobody laughed. Mrs. Miller shot him a glare that could have launched a few more rockets out to the moon.

"Never did have much imagination, that one," muttered Frank to himself.

Radio Addict

In 1964, nobody in town was more inseparable from their transistor radio than Pat “Radio” Reynolds. At 15, Pat had built his reputation on knowing every hit song, sports score, and weather report before anyone else. He even brought the radio to the dinner table—which drove his mom to the brink of confiscation. But Pat still kept his trusty transistor on him at all times, usually attached to his belt.

One Saturday afternoon, Pat and his buddies were at Johnny’s Diner when the jukebox broke down. Everyone turned to Pat’s radio to keep the tunes flowing while Johnny tried to fix the jukebox. But just as Pat was grooving to the latest Beatles hit, nature called.

“Sorry, fellas, can't let my 'little' guy out of my sight,” he joked, strapping the radio to his belt as he headed to the restroom.

Inside the restroom, Pat started humming along to the song, barely paying attention as he reached to adjust his belt. That's when it happened: the fateful *clink* and *splash*. In one tragic moment, Pat watched his precious radio flip out of his back pocket and straight into the toilet.

"Nooooo!" he dove into action like he was rescuing a drowning victim. At first, he bristled, his nose assaulted by the smell of the bowl before him. But then he took a deep breath and fished out the radio, horrified to see liquid dripping from every angle, so much so that he didn't even care that the liquid in question wasn't water. He shook it out, blew on it, and even whispered, "Come on, don't leave me now."

Nothing. The Beatles were gone. He might never get another weather forecast again.

When Pat returned with his soggy, silent, and slightly smelly radio, the guys took one look and burst out laughing. "Looks like the radio had to go too!" one of them cracked.

Tie-Dye Gone Wrong

In the summer of 1968, the tie-dye craze was in full swing, and nobody wanted to be the only kid without a swirling psychedelic wardrobe. So, one Saturday afternoon, I decided to take matters into my own hands and tie-dye half my closet. How hard could it be?

I gathered huge boxes of fabric dye, pails, rubber bands, and every white shirt of mine I could find. My mom had warned me not to make a mess, but with her gone to Aunt Margie's for the day, I figured I'd clean up before she returned. I even recruited my little brother Stan, who was mostly just there for the thrill of being involved in a "super duper top-secret project."

I filled the buckets with hot water and started pouring in every color of dye I had—bright blues, deep purples, neon greens. The pails were soon brimming and sloshing with swamps of color. I dunked in my clothes and twisted, tied, and swirled, grinning like a mad scientist.

Then it happened. I accidentally tilted the bucket of blue dye, and half of it spilled out onto the floor.

I panicked, and in the process, knocked over the buckets of dye next to it. Stan let out a shriek as purple and green rivers spread under the washer, oozed toward the door, and soaked our socks. When I involuntarily let go in horror, the blue dye followed suit and emptied itself onto the floor, too.

I desperately tried mopping it up with towels, which quickly turned psychedelic themselves. The floor was a neon horror scene, and I slipped on the slick rainbow mess, sending a dye-soaked towel flying. It hit poor Stan with a *splat*, leaving a bright blue splotch on his face.

When Mom came home, she found us scrubbing frantically as we left a trail of colorful handprints everywhere. After her initial gasp, she thankfully just laughed and shook her head. I became the tie-dye cautionary tale of the neighborhood and earned the moniker "Mister Dye-saster."

We Had a Band

In 1967, it felt like everyone had a band. The Beatles, the Stones—even some of the high school kids down the block were jamming out in their garages. I was convinced that the only thing standing between me and rockstar fame was getting a band together.

There was just one tiny problem: I couldn't play a *single* instrument.

But when has a lack of talent ever stopped anyone?

I roped in my best friends, Kenny, Ricky, and Paul. Kenny could sort of play guitar; Ricky's dad had an old drum kit collecting dust, and Paul had once taken a month of piano lessons. We were ready to blow the neighborhood away—as soon as I could figure out what to play.

I first tried bass, thinking, "How hard can four strings be?" But after a week of raw fingertips and only frog noises to show for it, I gave up. Then I tried drumming in place of Ricky. Only, a drumstick flew out of my hands and smacked Ricky in the face during a particularly intense practice. He never let me near the drums again after that!

My last hope was the harmonica; I would be the next Bob Dylan, only cooler. I bought one for two bucks at the drugstore and spent hours puffing away, hoping the neighbors didn't call animal control on me.

Finally, the day came for our debut at Paul's birthday party. As we started playing "Twist and Shout," I went all in on my harmonica solo. Unfortunately, I lost control of the harmonica; it flew out of my mouth, bounced off the amplifier, and went straight into the punch bowl.

The crowd went silent. Then, everyone burst out laughing. It wasn't the applause I'd dreamed of, but it was better than boos!

We disbanded shortly after that, but my legend as the "Robin Hood of harmonicas" lived on. The whole school talked about our show for weeks, but I decided to let my "musical talent" rest in peace.

Hippie Makeover

In 1969, Donnie Hoover was the very picture of "straight-laced." He had his hair neatly combed, shirts always tucked, and slacks pressed with a razor-sharp crease. But after a summer of Woodstock posters, groovy magazine covers, and tie-dye everywhere, Donnie decided he needed a change. He would join the counterculture—even if he had no clue what that really meant.

He started by growing his hair out—which actually meant he stopped brushing it for about three days before his mom practically threw a comb at him. Next, he borrowed a “Save the Earth” shirt from his hippie cousin, which came with an odd smell he tried not to think about. He even tried saying things like “far out” and “groovy,” although he made it sound like reciting Latin.

For the piece de resistance, he bought the most ridiculous bell-bottom pants he could find, paired them with a vest brimming with fringe tassels, and topped it all off with a rainbow bandana. He strolled into school on Monday feeling like a whole new person—or so he thought.

For one, he discovered he hadn’t bought bell-bottoms but some sort of odd knock-off flares that were too tight and too long. He tripped on the hem every few steps, face-planting on the hallway floor twice. A tassel on his vest got caught in the zipper of his backpack, resulting in an epic struggle that half the school watched as he wrestled with it like a crazed rodeo bull.

Then there was the bandana. No one had told him it was supposed to sit on his forehead—so he had tied it around his chin like a bonnet. People started calling him "Little Bo-Peep" behind his back. By lunch, even his friends were snickering, and the school’s “real” hippies couldn’t help but laugh. “Lookin' groovy, Donnie,” they teased.

Donnie eventually got the message, though; at the end of the day, he ditched the outfit, feeling like counterculture was just a little too... trippy for him.

Garter Trouble

In 1962, every girl who wanted to look classy wore nylons with a trusty garter belt to keep them up. Lora had just turned sixteen and was determined to look like an elegant adult, so when her mom finally let her wear nylons to the school dance, she was over the moon. She'd practiced with the garter belt all week, snapping it on and off with flair.

The night of the dance, Lora slipped into her new garter belt and secured her nylons as she'd practiced. They were pulled up snugly, garters clipped firmly, and she felt invincible. As she walked into the gym, she gave a little spin, her skirt twirling just enough to give a hint of her sophisticated hosiery. She noticed some boys glancing her way, and she couldn't help smiling.

Everything was going fine until about halfway through the night. She and her friends were dancing to a fast-tempo twist when she felt something strange. One of the garter straps had snapped off, dangling and tickling her leg. She ignored it, hoping it wouldn't be noticed, but just as she began to dance again, the second strap went.

Her nylons started rolling down like two rebellious snakes escaping her knees. Desperate, she tried shimmying them back up while dancing, but it was no use. A third snap and the last garter gave way, sending her nylons plummeting to her ankles in a mess.

In horror, she tried to play it off by shuffling her feet, but the sight of her bunched-up nylons and drooping garter belt was impossible to ignore. Her friend Sue nearly fell over laughing, and even the chaperone had to stifle a giggle. Lora's cheeks burned as red as her lipstick as she slinked to the bathroom to rip off the nylons and stuff them in her purse.

For a while after, Lora was known as "Garter Girl"; every time she'd pass by the boys, they'd give a dramatic tug on their imaginary nylons until she sheepishly shuffled away.

Twister

It was 1966, and Twister was the hottest game around. Every kid on our street wanted to test their flexibility and balance, and my cousin Timmy and I were no exception. We begged our parents to get the game for weeks, and they finally gave in on a rainy Saturday afternoon.

We rolled out the Twister mat in the living room, and soon, we had half the family twisting and contorting like human pretzels. Uncle Larry's knees were cracking, my mom was laughing so hard she nearly fell over, and Aunt Judy kept shouting directions that no one listened to. Then Grandpa, our referee, spun the wheel: “Left hand, green!”

I reached out, but just as I placed my hand on the green circle, there was a loud, tragic *rrriiiip*—right down the seam of my pants! I froze, realizing everyone had a front-row view of my plaid underwear. The whole family erupted in laughter, and I went beet red, trying to cover myself with my other hand while still balancing on the mat.

Just as I was about to crawl off and change, Grandpa suddenly had a change of heart. "I want to join in on the fun," he declared, his eyes twinkling. Despite our protests, he took my place on the mat, nearly squashing Aunt Judy’s foot while he was at it; Grandpa wasn’t the nimblest guy for his age. And then, just as he bent down to reach the next circle, we all heard it: a loud, unmistakable *pfffft*.

Everyone went silent, eyes wide, until Timmy burst into hysterics, practically rolling off the mat. Grandpa just chuckled. “It's only my joints letting off some steam!”

The rest of us tried to continue the game, but it was impossible. So we decided to stop, our stomachs hurting from laughing so hard at my split pants and Grandpa’s impromptu “trumpet solo.”

Bell-Bottom Biking

In 1969, bell-bottoms were everything. The bigger the flare, the cooler you were. So Ferris and Mike challenged each other to see who could have the widest bell-bottoms in the whole town. Every weekend, they'd stroll through the streets, giving dramatic spins so their pants could swoosh in all their glory. Mike's mom even sewed on extra fabric one week, and he showed up with flares so wide he looked like he was wearing two denim parachutes.

Not to be outdone, Ferris begged his mom to let him sew in more fabric, too. The result? He could barely squeeze out the front door without snagging a pant leg. But walking was one thing; biking would be another matter entirely.

One Saturday, Ferris decided to pedal over to Mike's house to show off his latest upgrade. He hopped on his bike, mega bell-bottoms catching the wind like sails. Ferris felt invincible—until he noticed his pants flapping dangerously close to the bike chain. But he shrugged it off, thinking he'd mastered his balance on two wheels.

Then disaster struck.

One enormous flare got sucked into the chain, and his bike screeched to a halt. Suddenly, Ferris was jerked forward, legs tangled, and he went down in a heap of fabric and metal. His bell-bottoms were wrapped around the chain like a python around its meal, and he was practically hog-tied to his bike.

As he struggled, Mike came riding down the street and burst out laughing when he saw Ferris sprawled out, voluminous bell-bottoms grease-stained and torn. “With bell-bottoms that wide, you should have taken a yacht!” he said, barely able to catch his breath.

By the time Ferris freed himself, he’d become a neighborhood spectacle. Kids pointed, moms shook their heads, and even old Mrs. Peabody chuckled as she walked by. Ferris decided to end his bell-bottom glory days right then. He resigned himself to watching Mike show off his flares—although, from that day on, even Mike would stay clear of any bicycles in the vicinity!

Minnie's Miniskirt

In 1967, Twiggy was the ultimate fashion icon. Every girl wanted to mimic that short miniskirt look—including Minnie, the least fashionable farm girl in town. She’d seen Twiggy’s photos in the magazines, her short skirts looking just too cool and glamorous. Against her mother’s warnings, Minnie decided to fashion her own miniskirt by cutting down an old dress to barely mid-thigh. She felt city-chic, ready to hit the fields in style.

The first test came after breakfast. Minnie had to feed the chickens, so she marched out, swinging a bucket of feed and feeling confident. But as soon as she crouched down, the skirt rode up to levels Twiggy herself might’ve thought twice about! Just as Minnie scrambled to pull it down, one of the hens pecked at her exposed legs, presumably confused by this new, brightly-colored “twiggy” creature in its coop. Minnie shrieked, and the whole flock scattered in a squawking frenzy, leaving feathers, feed, and Minnie's pride in tatters.

Next, Minnie had to help with the cows. Her mother warned that skirts and manure shoveling didn’t mix, but Minnie insisted, promising she'd be careful. But careful didn’t matter once she got into the barn.

As she leaned over to scoop some hay, a breeze blew through the barn, and the cows were gifted with a rather intimate view. Just then, Minnie's skirt caught on a nail sticking out of a stall door. She pulled back to free herself but instead slipped—and fell straight into a fresh pile of manure.

By lunchtime, Minnie was covered in feathers, mud, and a questionable scent that had the family dog sniffing her suspiciously. Her mother took one look at the ruined miniskirt and shook her head.

“Twiggy might have style, Minnie, but she doesn’t have farm chores,” she chuckled.

Minnie retreated back to her room and quickly swapped back to her usual practical clothes. When she strode back out again in her well-worn jeans, so ended the brief yet dramatic saga of the "Minnie-Skirt."

Crack the Whip

In 1964, winter meant one thing: ice skating on the frozen pond. And for eleven-year-old Oscar, this winter was his big chance to skate with his older brother Danny and his friends, who ruled the pond as they zoomed around with ease. They'd play "crack the whip," linking hands in a chain and flinging the last kid at breakneck speed. Oscar was desperate to try it, though he'd only just mastered skating without clinging to a friend for balance.

One Saturday, he finally worked up the nerve to ask, "Hey, can I play?"

Danny raised an eyebrow but shrugged. "Sure, little dude. Just hold on tight."

Oscar lined up, heart thumping as he grabbed Danny's hand and clung to a bigger kid on his other side. The line stretched across the ice, and they started slowly, swinging in a wide arc.

But the speed picked up. Suddenly, he was sliding so fast he barely felt the ice under his feet. The chain whipped around, and the pond's snowy banks became a blur. Oscar's mouth dropped open, equal parts thrilled and terrified.

Then Danny shouted, "Hold on, we're gonna crack it!"

The whole line jerked, and Oscar felt himself flying outwards as the whip cracked. His hand slipped, and before he could even shout, he was launched off the end of the whip like a human slingshot. Arms and legs flailing, he flew through the air and landed butt-first in a huge snowbank on the edge of the pond, legs sticking out in a wobbly "V."

The big kids were doubled over with laughter, skating over to pull him out. Even Danny had to laugh when he saw Oscar's snow-covered head.

"You okay, little dude?" he chuckled.

Oscar shook off the snow, grinning ear-to-ear despite his bruised pride and even more bruised bum. "Yeah... let's go again!"

Danny snorted. "Alright, but your butt's going to regret it tomorrow."

Oscar began to understand what that meant after his fourth flight into the snowbank.

The Twist

In 1961, everyone in our generation was doing The Twist. Chubby Checker was blaring from every radio, and the kids were swiveling and twisting so hard you'd think they were trying to drill themselves into the ground. My friend Judy and I practiced the dance every chance we got.

One Saturday night, the town hall hosted a sock hop, and it seemed like the perfect opportunity to debut our moves to a bigger audience. Judy and I planned to hit the dance floor the second we heard the opening beat of The

Twist. We assumed the older folks would stay on the sidelines with their punch cups, watching politely or cheering on. We didn't consider the fact that they might have, well, *mixed* opinions—and loud ones at that!

As soon as the DJ dropped the needle on The Twist, Judy and I flung ourselves onto the dance floor, twisting and wiggling with all our might. More kids joined in, and soon, the place was packed with twisters, everyone swiveling and spinning in one big, chaotic mass. We thought we looked pretty cool—but the grown-ups stared at us in shock.

Mrs. Flanders, who usually sold raffle tickets, clutched her pearls and gasped. "They look like they're wringing out a bunch of wet towels!"

Mr. Brentwood, who ran the hardware store, shook his head, squinting at us like we were possessed by demons. "Is that... dancing?" he asked. "Looks more like they're trying to wiggle out of their own skin!"

At one point, old Jack Reagan shuffled over toward the dance floor with his demure wife, Gladys. He watched for a moment, then declared loudly, "In my day, we held our partners when we danced!" He tried to show us, grabbing Gladys and doing a little ballroom step—until his back cracked and his knees popped so loudly they nearly drowned out Chubby Checker! With a feeble grunt, he was escorted back out again by Gladys, while us younger kids held back giggles and resumed our "unholy gyrations."

Not-So-Chatty Cathy

In 1963, Ethel Kellogg got a Chatty Cathy doll for Christmas. The doll came with a string that could be pulled, and she'd then say things like, "I love you!" or "Let's play!" The toy was adorable... until Ethel got her hands on it.

Ethel was only six, but she was a budding little scientist, always curious about how things worked. Naturally, Cathy's voice box became her prime experiment. One afternoon, Ethel's older sister Lorna walked into the bedroom to find Ethel with Cathy flipped over, toy screwdrivers and other tools scattered across the floor. She looked up, grinning like a tiny mad scientist.

"What are you doing to Chatty Cathy?" Lorna was wide-eyed.

"I'm makin' her talk more!" Ethel declared proudly. Then she yanked Cathy's string as hard as she could and then... nothing. Cathy was silent.

Ethel blinked at the doll, frowning. "Chatty Cathy? Say something!" She pulled the string again, and Cathy let out a scratchy noise that sounded like a ghost with a sore throat.

Ethel's eyes went wide, but she didn't give up. She wound the string tighter, and this time Cathy managed a haunting "Loooove yoouuuu..." that sent shivers down the spine. It sounded like Cathy had developed a severe case of "possessed doll."

Ethel nervously yanked the string one more time; Cathy suddenly blurted out, “Let’s plaaaayyyyyy… play… play…” in a stretched-out echo that made Ethel drop her in shock. The doll just lay there, sputtering out a few more garbled phrases before falling silent again, seemingly for good. In a panic, Lorna kicked her under the bed.

Chatty Cathy was left there to rest, with Lorna and Ethel too afraid to touch her again. But sometimes at night, they’d hear a faint, glitchy “I looooove yooouuu” coming from under the bed and would hug each other in fright. It wasn't all bad, though—Ethel focused on her studies more so she'd never make the same mistake with another toy again!

Troll Dolls

In 1967, troll dolls were all the rage, with their wild neon hair and goofy grins. Ian's friends each had one and soon dove into a fierce competition: who could give their troll the best name? A troll doll with a lame name just wasn’t as cool.

Ian started off rather basic. His troll had bright orange hair, so Ian named him "Blaze." But his friend Susie came in strong with “Prince Bongo.” She’d made him a crown out of aluminum foil and had placed little cork bongos at his hands for added flair. That was when everyone began to up their game.

The next day, Ian showed up with Blaze upgraded to "Sir Blazington." He'd drawn a tiny mustache on him with a permanent marker, convinced this made him look like nobility. But then Bobby came by with his troll, which he named "Thunderfuzz, Troll of Thunder." Thunderfuzz had hair that was teased to the heavens and glued so stiff it looked like he'd stuck his finger in a socket.

The naming contest quickly escalated. Every recess was spent showing off their trolls' new personalities. Jenny's troll became "Madame Stardust," with glitter covering her entire head. Carla went full hippie and named her troll "Cosmic Moonbeam," braiding its hair with beads and dressing it in tiny bell-bottoms.

Finally, Ian returned with yet another set of upgrades to his troll, which included a wobbly round crown that almost resembled a bum and a fiery red gown. He dramatically set it on the table and declared, "I present... His Royal Highness, King Wigglebottom Blazington the Third!"

The name sent everyone into hysterics. "King Wigglebottom Blazington the Third" had officially won the naming competition, hands down. No one could top it. Even the teacher cracked a smile when she heard it. And so it was that King Wigglebottom reigned supreme over his troll domain.

Sunday Best and White Gloves

In 1965, Sunday mornings were no joke in our family. My mom had us dressed to the nines for church—pressed suits for the boys and frilly dresses, hats, and white gloves for the girls. This was serious business. One particular Sunday, though, things were a little... unorthodox.

Mom had spent the whole night ironing and preparing our Sunday best, and by morning, the house was a flurry of buttoning, polishing, and brushing. I had a brand-new pink dress with puffed sleeves and a giant bow in the back, which made me feel like gift-wrapped cotton candy. Meanwhile, my brother Tommy constantly struggled to get his clip-on tie straight, grumbling under his breath the whole time.

By the time we piled into the station wagon, we were somehow early, which was nothing short of a miracle. But then Mom let out a gasp. "My gloves! Where are my gloves?" She scrambled through her purse, but they were nowhere to be found. "Everyone, back inside! We'll find them quick!"

So we raced back inside, took off our shoes, and tore through drawers, the closet, the laundry basket, and even the dog's bed. Mom finally found her gloves under the couch, and we flew back into the car and zoomed off.

We barely made it to church on time—yet another miracle! Mom hurried us in, her white gloves on and her hat perfectly tilted. But as we took our seats, a few heads turned and some eyebrows rose. I glanced down and realized… in our mad dash back out of the house, I had put on mismatched shoes! I looked over, and Tommy's clip-on tie was upside down and dangling crooked as well. Mom’s dress had little fuzz balls still clinging to it from the glove hunt, looking less “Sunday best” and more “dust bunny chic.”

Dad managed to find the humor in our situation, though. "I guess this is the opposite of being fashionably late—being unfashionably on time!"

Pill Box

In the summer of 1962, Gloria was obsessed with pillbox hats. Jackie Kennedy and Doris Day both wore them with such glamorous style that Gloria dreamed of having her own. So when she found a perfect, pale-blue pillbox at the local department store, she just had to have it, despite her husband Barry’s half-hearted warning that it was pricey for a hat that "doesn’t even cover your head."

A week later, they went with some friends to the county fair. Gloria was two months along in her first pregnancy, and while she didn’t have much of a bump, she was already battling morning sickness—which apparently cared very little for the actual time of day! But nothing would stop her from showing off her new hat.

As they strolled through the fair, Gloria held her head high, the pillbox firmly secured with two bobby pins and a lot of confidence. She looked like a picture out of Good Housekeeping until they got to the Tilt-A-Whirl. Barry suggested she sit out, but Gloria wasn't about to miss out on the fun. So, pillbox hat and all, she climbed aboard.

She would regret it soon enough.

Halfway through the ride, her face turned an impressive shade of green. She held on tightly, trying to focus on anything other than the churning in her stomach, but it was no use. When the inevitable happened, she frantically reached for anything she could use. And so off came the prized pillbox hat in a tragic twist, becoming an emergency barf bag.

The ride stopped, and Gloria stumbled off, holding her suddenly un-glamorous pillbox at arm's length, face flushed and eyes wide. Her friends tried to stifle their laughter while she stood there mortified, Barry sympathetically patting her shoulder.

Despite how much it had cost, Gloria was quick to chuck the odorous pillbox into the nearest bin at the fair. As she walked away, she sighed. "I wonder if Jackie ever did this?"

Mop Tops and Meltdowns

In 1964, every kid on the block wanted a Beatles haircut, and Jonah was no different. He was convinced that if he could get that perfect mop-top like Paul McCartney, he'd be the coolest kid in fifth grade. After weeks of begging, his mom finally caved and agreed to take him to a local barber who "knew all the new styles."

Mr. Tony, the barber, was more used to giving buzz cuts and flat tops, but he nodded seriously when Jonah said he wanted "a mop top like a Beatle." Mr. Tony didn't actually know what a Beatles haircut was, but he knew something about tops. "You got it, kid," he said, snapping his scissors confidently.

Jonah's mom waited in the front during the haircut, flipping through a magazine. Mr. Tony started snipping away, and Jonah watched huge clumps of his hair fall to the floor. He didn't know much about haircuts, but he began to worry when his bangs were cut short. "Um, Mr. Tony, are you sure this is—?"

Mr. Tony cut him off. "Trust me, kiddo."

Finally, Jonah was spun around to face the mirror, and his jaw dropped. Instead of a soft mop, he had an unholy mix of a flat top with a bowl cut. With his spindly hair, he looked more like a scared hedgehog than Paul McCartney.

He stumbled out of the chair, his mom stifling a gasp, while an oblivious Mr. Tony beamed proudly. "There ya go! One 'Beatles' flat top." He didn't even wince when Jonah's mother furiously explained that they'd wanted a 'mop' top instead.

Back home and on the verge of a meltdown, Jonah desperately tried to tame the mess. But when he combed it down with water, it looked less like a mop top—and more like an actual mop head.

Grandma and Go-Go Boots

In 1968, Grandma decided she wanted to "get with the times." She'd seen all the young gals on TV rocking miniskirts and those white, knee-high Go-Go boots. While she wouldn't dare try a miniskirt, she made my mom take her to the mall to find herself a pair of Go-Go boots.

We all thought it was just talk until she came home, grinning ear-to-ear and wobbling through the front door in a brand-new pair of glossy white boots. They hugged her legs like sausage casings, but Grandma didn't care. "Aren't they something?" she said, doing a shaky twirl in the kitchen. We had to admit, she at least had spunk!

Days later, Grandma insisted on wearing her new boots for a big family trip to the department store. As we headed to the escalator, she marched ahead of us, strutting like she was in a fashion show.

But halfway down, Grandma's foot slipped—and one boot heel got caught in the edge of the escalator step! She yelped, stumbling as she tried to pull her foot free, but the escalator had a fierce grip. The boot was stuck, and with each clanking step, it yanked her foot back like some mechanical monster.

"Stop the escalator! It's eating my foot!" she shrieked, clutching the handrail for dear life.

My dad ran to find a store clerk while Mom held Grandma's arm, trying to calm her down. Meanwhile, Grandma's other foot was flying every which way as she tried to wiggle her boot free. A small crowd gathered, half of them concerned, the other half trying not to laugh.

Thankfully, a young employee stopped the escalator in time and freed Grandma's boot with a crowbar. She emerged injury-free, but her prized white boot was now streaked with black grease, while the other was scuffed all over from her earlier panic. Grandma looked at them, sighed, and said, "Well, I guess these boots are going to have to go-go."

The 1970s

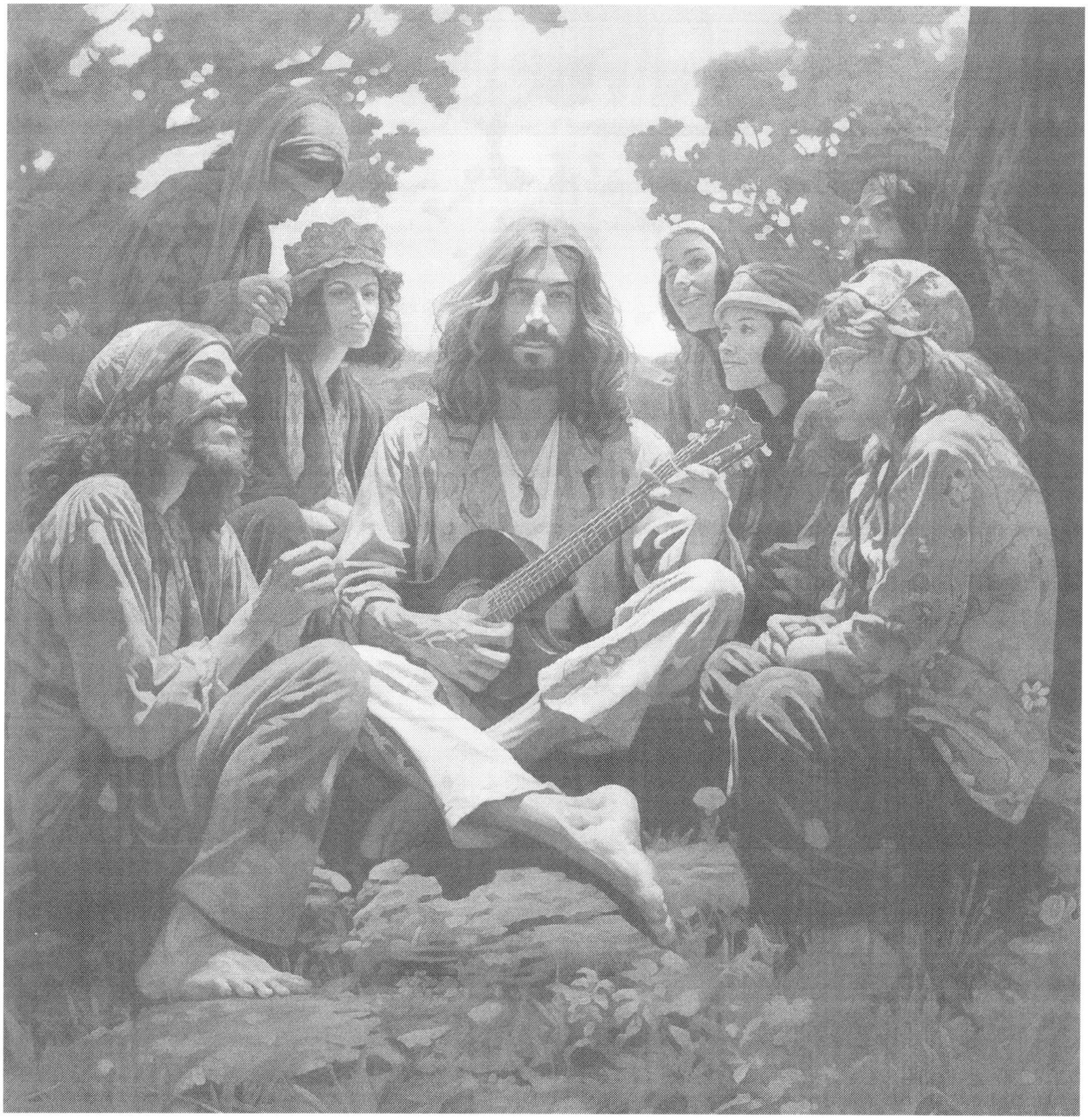

Shag Rug Shambles

In 1976, sixteen-year-old Linda was thrilled to earn her first babysitting gig for the Andersons, a cool family with bean bag chairs and a sprawling, lime-green shag rug that felt like walking on a thick field of grass. They went out for dinner, leaving her to watch over their six-year-old son Fred.

Things were going smoothly until Fred wanted dinner, so Linda made him a bowl of cereal and marshmallows. Fred decided it would be hilarious to knock the whole thing over onto the shag carpet—food everywhere, wedged deep into the long green fibers.

Linda panicked. But then she thought, *Just vacuum it up, silly!* So she wheeled out the Andersons' crimson Hoover, flipped the power switch, and set the vacuum's beater attachment onto the spill. The vacuum roared to life—but so did the shag carpet! Carpet strands began to wrap around the beater brush, tangling up in an epic carpet-versus-vacuum showdown. Linda was horrified as the vacuum started to smell like burning rubber and made a noise like a growling guard dog.

Linda anxiously yanked the vacuum back, but it was too late—the shag rug was firmly latched onto the beater. She knelt down and tried to pry the fibers free, but her fingers kept getting tangled. Fred, watching this disaster unfold, started laughing. She was elbow-deep in shag and vacuum when she heard the front door creak open.

In walked Mrs. Anderson, a mix of confusion and amusement spreading across her face as she took in the sight: Linda crouched on the shag rug in a battle with the vacuum, surrounded by cereal, and Fred laughing his head off.

"Oh, Mrs. Anderson!" Linda squeaked, her hand still clamped around a rogue tangle of shag carpet. "I was just fixing up a snack for Fred, and this happened."

Mrs. Anderson raised an eyebrow. "You didn't have to also feed the Hoover, dear."

Disco Disaster

It was 1978, and Charlie had discovered the magic of disco. Every Friday night, his friends would hit up the roller rink, and Charlie would dazzle them with his moves—at least, so he thought. Charlie's mom, however, wasn't thrilled with him practicing "that flashy dance" in the living room, especially since he had a history of clumsiness and the living room was packed with delicate knickknacks.

One Saturday night, Charlie's parents were out, and he had the house to himself. He cranked up his record player, and *Stayin' Alive* by the Bee Gees boomed through the room. Dressed in a polyester shirt with an open collar, a massive belt buckle, and bell-bottoms, Charlie was ready to bring some disco spirit to suburbia.

Feeling the groove, he spun, swiveled, and got down low, every finger-point in sync with the beat. He launched with flair into his grand finale—the Hustle.

But on the third backward step, Charlie lost control. His flared pants snagged on the carpet, throwing off his balance. In a flurry of polyester and flailing arms, he crashed directly into his mom's favorite coffee table.

The table made a terrible crack, and the bowl of plastic fruit on it went flying. In one horrifying, slow-motion moment, Charlie watched as two apples, some bananas, and a sad-looking bunch of grapes bounced across the room and landed with thuds. He hit the floor with a *whoof*, clutching his toe in pain.

And then his parents walked in.

They stopped in the doorway, taking in the scene: Charlie, sprawled on the floor in bell-bottoms and clutching his foot, the coffee table listing dramatically to one side, and plastic fruit littering the carpet. Charlie's mom gasped, while his dad just shook his head. "Disco? More like 'Dis Go' badly!"

8-Track Tangle

It was 1977, and Glen had just bought *Rumours* by Fleetwood Mac on 8-track, using all the money he'd saved from mowing lawns. He was obsessed with the album, playing it constantly in his dad's beat-up Ford Pinto. As soon as he turned the key, *Go Your Own Way* blasted through the crackly speakers, and Glen felt like the coolest guy in town.

One Friday night, after picking up his buddies for a drive around town, Glen slid the tape into the player. But this time, instead of hearing Stevie Nicks' smoky voice, he was met with a terrible, garbled screech. The music slowed down to a strange, eerie drawl, and then... silence.

Glen's heart sank. He tried ejecting the tape, but it wouldn't budge. "C'mon, c'mon!" he muttered, frantically pressing buttons, but nothing worked. Finally, he gave the tape a good yank—and out came the 8-track, along with what looked like a mile of tangled tape spilling everywhere.

His friends gasped in amusement as Glen sat there horrified, staring at his ruined Fleetwood Mac masterpiece. Determined to save his beloved album, Glen started carefully pulling and rewinding the tape back into the cartridge. He licked his fingers, squinted, and twisted each bit of tape as if he were performing delicate surgery.

"Dude, just buy a new one." His friend Mike snickered.

"Do you know how much I paid for this?" Glen shot back, not willing to let *Rumours* go down without a fight.

After a few painstaking minutes, Glen managed to stuff the tape back into the cartridge. He shoved it into the player, crossed his fingers, and turned the volume up. Miraculously, it started playing again—for a few seconds. Then the tape gave one last gargle and shredded itself with a gut-wrenching snap.

Just then, a car full of girls pulled alongside them, windows down, looking curiously as they heard the sputtering of Glen's ruined 8-track. He could only sigh as Mike hollered, "Don't worry, ladies, it's just Fleetwood Mac—they're really going their own way!"

Lava Lamp Eruption

It was 1975, and my room was the ultimate '70s paradise: shag carpet, posters of Led Zeppelin, and, of course, my pride and joy—a bright red lava lamp. I'd saved up for weeks to buy that baby, and it was mesmerizing. I'd sit there for hours, watching the blobs of wax float up and down; it was the coolest thing ever!

One Saturday night, my friend Dave came over to listen to records. I decided to crank up *Smoke on the Water* and set the lava lamp right next to my speakers so the blobs would "dance" to the beat. We were totally into it, feeling like we were front-row at a Deep Purple concert.

But then, halfway through the song, we noticed the lava blobs were moving a little *too* wildly.

"Hey, is it supposed to do that?" Dave pointed at the lamp, where the blobs of wax were bubbling up fast and furiously. I shrugged, thinking it was just the lava lamp's way of feeling the music.

Then, with a sudden, terrifying *BLOP*, the top of the lava lamp blew off, and thick, goopy red wax shot straight up and splattered across the ceiling. Dave and I screamed and ducked as if we were under attack. Globs of hot wax rained down on my bed, my Zeppelin poster, and my prized shag carpet.

Dave was rolling on the floor, somehow finding it funny, while I frantically grabbed tissues, a sock—anything—to wipe up the mess. "Dude, your mom is going to kill you!" he gasped between hysterics. I looked around in horror, realizing he was right.

As if on cue, my mom poked her head in, her jaw dropping as she took in the ceiling, the carpet, and my red-splattered face.

There was no hiding this eruption.

Madelyn's Disco Fever

It was 1978, and Madelyn had been dying to check out the new disco club in town, Groove Central. She'd seen *Saturday Night Fever* at least ten times and had spent hours perfecting her finger-pointing and hip-swaying moves in front of her bedroom mirror. She was convinced she'd dazzle the crowd.

One Saturday night, she finally made it to Groove Central with her friends. The place was everything she'd dreamed of—mirror balls, flashing lights, and *Le Freak* by Chic blaring through the speakers. Dressed in a sparkly jumpsuit and sky-high platform shoes, she was ready to become a disco queen. As soon as they hit the dance floor, Madelyn struck a dramatic pose and launched into the Hustle.

Her friends tried to keep up, but Madelyn was unstoppable. She spun, she dipped, and she even attempted a daring move she'd seen John Travolta pull off—a swift slide-back with one leg extended.

Unfortunately, in her excitement, she didn't account for the slippery floor, her four-inch platforms—or the fact that she'd only practiced this move in socks on a shag carpet.

Mid-slide, her foot shot out from under her, and with a yelp, she tumbled backward, arms flailing wildly. In a flash, she saw herself reflected in every glittering disco ball above as she fell. She hit the floor with a spectacular crash, one leg bent at a painful angle, and an epic sound that silenced the entire dance floor; even the DJ stopped the music out of concern.

Her friends rushed over, but she couldn't get up; her ankle had twisted something fierce. Mortified and trying to hold onto her pride, Madelyn was carried out of Groove Central and straight to the ER, her jumpsuit torn and her platforms dangling from her hands.

The ER nurse had an eyebrow raised. "So, what happened?"

Madelyn sighed, feeling her cheeks burn as her friends filled the nurse in on the details.

The nurse smiled. "Sounds like you caught a bad case of Disco Fever, dear."

Hustle Up Mom

In 1977, Mom became obsessed with disco. She'd seen *Saturday Night Fever,* and therefore thought she was destined to become the next disco queen. One night after dinner, she announced, "Alright, kids, it's time you teach me how to do the Hustle!"

My brother Jimmy and I exchanged horrified glances. Mom was more of a polka lady who broke out her accordion at family gatherings. Disco... was a stretch.

“Oh, c’mon,” she insisted, waving her hands in what she thought was a groovy dance move. “You two are always dancing around. Show your old mom a thing or two!”

Reluctantly, we cleared the living room. Mom had pulled on her “fancy” bell-bottoms and a sequined vest she’d dug out from her college days, her hair teased into a dramatic beehive that added a solid three inches to her height. She somehow looked like a disco diva and a 1950s housewife at the same time.

“Alright, so you start with the basic moves,” Jimmy demonstrated. Mom tried to copy, pointing her fingers and stepping side to side, but her timing was hilariously off. She either rushed ahead, halfway across the room, or fell behind, crashing into the couch.

“Faster, faster!” she demanded, so Jimmy and I sped up, hoping she’d give up. Instead, she started spinning wildly, trying to keep up, flinging her arms and making up moves of her own, which looked like a mutant child of Disco and the Twist.

Then came her grand finale: She attempted the famous finger-point spin, but her beehive caught on the light fixture above. For a split second, she was stuck, bobbing back and forth as she tried to free her hair. With a final yank, she broke free, but her momentum sent her stumbling right into the couch, sending a cushion flying in the process.

We rushed over to check if she was alright; she was sprawled out and red-faced but laughing cheerfully. "Well, if nothing else, all this hustling is a good workout!”

The Streaking Incident

In 1974, streaking was suddenly the trending "crazy" thing you could do—or at least that’s what my friend Andy thought. He’d seen streakers on TV at baseball games, on college campuses, even at the Grammys. So, naturally, Andy got it in his head that he was destined to make his mark with his own epic streaking incident.

One Saturday afternoon, we were hanging out at the local mall. The place was packed with shoppers, families, and teenagers looking to spend their allowance. Andy took a deep breath, turned to me, and said, “Hold my clothes.” Before I could even process what he meant, he’d stripped down to his pale bare bottom, handed me his clothes, and took off, bare-chested, running right through the main atrium of the mall.

At first, nobody noticed. But once Andy started hooting and hollering, he quickly became the center of attention. Shoppers stopped in their tracks, jaws dropping as he zigzagged around the fountains, past the Orange Julius, and down the hall toward the food court.

"Andy, are you crazy?" I shouted after him, holding his clothes awkwardly.

By the time he hit the food court, security guards were hot on his trail. Andy spotted them and took them on a wild goose chase through the mall. He thought he had them when he saw and sprinted toward the nearest exit—only to realize that the door led to a convenience store. He dashed in, nearly knocking over a rack of postcards and causing an elderly lady to scream in shock.

Unfortunately for Andy, the convenience store was a dead end. Cornered by security and watched by a group of Girl Scouts with their mouths hanging open, he had no choice but to surrender. The guards tried not to laugh as they escorted him out.

As for me? I left as discreetly as I could. On the way out, I saw Andy's mom coming in, so I gave her his clothes and ran before she could recover from the shock enough to grill me!

CB Antics

In 1976, Toby got a CB radio for his birthday, and he became obsessed with it. Toby was convinced he was now part of some secret trucker brotherhood, even though he was only sixteen and the only thing he'd ever driven was his dad's lawnmower. He spent hours picking out his "handle" (he went with "Hot

Wheels") and practicing his best trucker voice, which sounded like Clint Eastwood with a cold.

One weekend, he dragged his cousin Linus out to his dad's garage to "hit the airwaves" with him. Toby was on a mission to talk to real truckers, and he thought I'd be his perfect sidekick. He even gave Linus a handle: "Sidecar Sally." Linus wasn't given a chance to object.

They sat there in a musty Buick, Toby fumbling with the CB radio controls, making static-y noises as he tried to reach the truckers. "Breaker one-nine, this is Hot Wheels," he called, puffing out his chest. "Any good buddies out there?"

At first, it was just static. Then, out of nowhere, a gravelly voice came through. "This is Big Bear, whatcha got, Hot Wheels?"

Toby's eyes lit up. He got so excited he started rambling nonsense about the "road conditions" on Main Street (where the Buick was parked) and asking Big Bear for "tips on hauling heavy loads" (the Buick only had some soccer gear in the trunk).

Toby was so caught up with his antics that Linus had to practically smack him over the head to get his attention. "Hey, what gives?" Linus simply pointed at the street—and the massive truck that had popped up right outside their house.

When Toby saw his mom determinedly head their way after talking to the grizzly looking driver of the truck, he frantically tried to open the door and make a run for it. But he was seconds too late.

"Toby, that nice young man over there says he's 'Big Bear' and is looking for some poor fella in need called... 'Hot Wheels'?"

Grandma's Crochet Vests

In 1975, Grandma Marcie discovered the first of two big passions: crochet. Her new mission became covering the entire family (starting with her grandkids) in her "masterpieces." Every time they visited, Grandma would have a new pile of crochet projects waiting, each one more stylish than the last—or so she believed!

It started with vests. She crocheted them in every color of the rainbow, complete with frills, pom-poms, and even tassels. She'd measure her grandkids meticulously, muttering things like, "Oh, just wait until your friends at school see these beauties!" Little Billy got a neon orange vest with big floppy pockets, and his older sister Sarah was gifted a bright green one with a fringe that went down to her knees. Their cousin Winslow got a sky-blue one with a giant sunflower in the middle.

Wearing those vests outside of Grandma's house was torture. Billy, Sarah, and Winslow were christened "the Flower Power Kids," and one kid in the neighborhood asked if they were "part of some hippie band."

It couldn't have gotten much worse... until Grandma discovered macramé.

One weekend, the entire living room was draped in knotted ropes. Plant hangers hung from every corner, and macramé art covered her walls. And Grandma had a gleam in her eye. "Guess what, kids? I'm making macramé ponchos for all of you!"

That Christmas, they each got a customized macramé poncho, complete with long fringes that nearly brushed the floor. Winslow's had seashells woven into the fringe, and Sarah's had chunky wooden beads that clacked whenever she moved. Billy's had a giant owl face on the back, and he felt like it was constantly watching him.

They wore those ponchos for exactly one family photo, everyone stiff and grimacing, while Grandma beamed proudly behind them. Later, the ponchos were quietly stuffed into the attic, never to see the light of day again. And from that day on, the kids loudly groaned whenever Grandma Marcie showed signs of picking up a new hobby.

Mood Rings

In 1978, mood rings were the hottest trend, and every kid at school had one. When Nicole finally got her own, she was convinced it could read her every thought and feeling. She spent a weekend watching it change colors, sure that every shift was revealing some new insight into her personality.

The next Monday, she proudly wore the mood ring to school, eager to show it off. Her friends crowded around, gasping as it changed from green to blue to purple, all consulting the tiny mood chart that came with it. "Green means you're relaxed," Lisa declared. "And purple... Well, that means you're feeling mysterious."

At that moment, Nicole sneezed, which ruined the mystery just a bit.

By lunchtime, the mood ring was a murky grayish-brown, which wasn't even on the chart. "Uh-oh," Tony said, inspecting it with a frown. "I think that means you're stressed. Or... maybe mad?" Suddenly, Nicole was second-guessing everything. *Was she mad? At who? Did she look stressed?* The ring's color simply grew murkier.

The real disaster happened when Nicole was late to math class. Mrs. Duncan, who was serious on a good day, noticed the mood ring and leaned in to look; right as she did, the ring turned a brilliant, fiery red. Mrs. Duncan raised an eyebrow and crossed her arms. “I see,” she said. “This ring thinks you’re feeling… passionate?”

“Oh, no, Mrs. Duncan!” Nicole stammered. “It’s broken. Or maybe it just, uh, doesn’t like Mondays?” Mrs. Duncan gave her extra homework since she was apparently so taken up with the subject.

By the time Nicole got home, the ring was still red, which she decided really meant “embarrassed and fuming.” Then her mother glanced at it and commented drily, "Thinking of boys again, are you, Nicole?" So, of course, her little sister got in on the act and teased Nicole until her face matched the red on her ring.

Waterbeds and Wobbles

In 1976, my parents bought a waterbed. It was the latest craze, and they proudly declared it would be like sleeping on a cloud. My dad spent all weekend setting it up, filling it with water and marveling at how futuristic it was. So, of course, I begged them to let me try it, and after enough pleading, they finally agreed to let me sleep on it for one night.

Climbing onto the waterbed felt like trying to stand on a giant jelly mold. I immediately sank in, the bed wobbling and sloshing beneath me. It was thrilling at first, though, like a private wave pool just for sleeping. I stretched out, feeling pretty smug that I'd managed to score a night on this marvel.

The trouble started when I tried to turn over. I rolled to my side, and the waterbed bucked and heaved as if I'd just caused an earthquake. The motion kept going, waves crashing up and down until I felt like I was on a rollercoaster. Every slight movement seemed to set off another wave, and soon, I was feeling seasick. I didn't even know that was possible in bed!

Just when I thought I had it under control, I decided to sit up for a glass of water from the bedside table—bad move. The moment I lifted the glass, the bed started sloshing wildly again, tilting me backward like I was on a runaway canoe. My glass of water spilled everywhere, which only added to the disaster. I thrashed around, trying to sit on the thin wooden frame around the bed, which just made the waves worse. I eventually slipped off the frame entirely, landing on the floor in a dizzy heap.

The next morning, I hobbled into the kitchen, looking like I'd been through a storm at sea. My dad grinned knowingly. "How'd it go last night?"

"Great," I muttered, rubbing my back. "I slept like a log—on the floor!"

Sneaking and Corduroys

In 1979, Gordon learned the hard way that corduroy pants and sneaking don't mix. He'd been out at his friend Mike's party, which ran a little later—and a little louder—than he'd told his parents it would. By the time he got home, the house was pitch dark, and he figured his parents were asleep. If he could just tiptoe in, he'd make it to his room without a sound.

Except...

Gordon was wearing his favorite corduroy pants: thick, ketchup-red, wide-wale corduroys. Normally, he loved them; they were his "swanky" pants, he stood out in them, and they swished when he walked, which he thought was awesome. But not for long.

As he stepped into the house, he took one cautious stride. *Swish-SWISH*. He winced. In the dark and empty interior, it sounded like someone was sawing wood with every step. He tried to take smaller steps, but somehow, this just made it worse. *SWISH-swish, SWISH-swish*. It echoed in the silence of the hallway.

He froze, cringing, convinced he'd woken the entire neighborhood. Taking a deep breath, he decided to go for it—one long, bold stride after another. *SWISH SWISH SWISH SWISH*. He moved as quickly as he could, hoping his parents would think it was just the wind or... something.

Just as he reached the living room, he heard a voice. "Gordon? Is that you?"

The lamp on the coffee table revealed his mom sitting in her recliner with a cup of tea, smirking like she'd been waiting for him all night. His dad was right behind her, looking both amused and exasperated.

"Nice try," his dad said, crossing his arms. "We could hear you swishing from the driveway."

Gordon's face turned as red as his bell-bottoms. He tried to explain about the party, but every attempt was met with another round of laughter. From then on, his parents called those corduroys his "sneaky pants"—and Gordon made sure they stayed well and truly hidden from sight!

Platform Shoe Peril

In 1977, Helen Boykins fell in love with a pair of sky-high platform shoes. She'd saved up all her babysitting money to buy them—silver, sparkly, and with a six-inch heel that she was convinced would make her look just like a disco queen. She strutted around the house in them, towering over everyone, and said she was "finally tall enough to command a room."

The first big test came that Saturday when she decided to wear them to the mall with her friends. She insisted on practicing her walk for hours before they left, clomping up and down the living room like a disco Frankenstein. Mrs.

Boykins warned her that those shoes weren't made for serious walking, but Helen just rolled her eyes. "Mom, I know what I'm doing."

So off they went to the mall. At first, Helen managed fine, tottering along with a confidence that bordered on recklessness. She was actually starting to get looks from strangers, and she whispered to her friends, "See? Everyone's staring because I'm fabulous."

But things took a sharp turn—literally—when they got to the food court. Helen spotted a cute guy at the hotdog stand and decided to give him her best strut. She turned, flipped her hair, and took one big, dramatic step. But with those platforms, her foot rolled right off the side, twisting her ankle and sending her lurching forward like a tower collapsing. She tried to steady herself, but the shoes wobbled, and down she went, arms flailing, directly into the condiment cart.

Ketchup, mustard, and relish flew everywhere, splattering her silver shoes and sparkly outfit. Her friends stared in shock as she sat there, legs sprawled out, with a mustard stain on one shoe and ketchup dripping down her shin.

The worst part, though, was that the cute guy simply burst out laughing.

This was probably the main reason why, when she hobbled home that night, she chucked the shoes into a bin and declared, "Platforms are a menace!"

The Great Microwave Popcorn Incident

In 1975, our family got our first microwave, and it was like having a piece of space-age technology right in our kitchen. Dad was fascinated, reading the instruction manual cover to cover, though none of us knew exactly what to do with it yet. One night, he decided we'd try out the ultimate test: microwave popcorn. He'd heard people raving about how quick and easy it was, and he figured it'd be a breeze. Little did we know we were in for The Great Microwave Popcorn Incident of '75.

Dad set the bag in the microwave, proudly pressing the buttons as if he were launching a rocket. "This should only take a few minutes," he winked at us. My sister and I watched in awe, waiting for the magic to begin. Sure enough, we started hearing pops, soft at first, then louder and faster. The bag was puffing up, filling with glorious buttery popcorn.

But something didn't seem quite right. The pops grew faster, louder, almost violent. The bag expanded until it looked practically glued to the microwave walls. Dad frowned. "Maybe that's just part of the—"

Boom!

The bag burst open, popcorn exploding everywhere inside the microwave like a firework.

When Dad opened the door, a mountain of popcorn spilled out and completely covered his feet. He stood there stunned as kernels continued to pop and spill across the counter. Our dog started barking, thinking it was some new kind of treat, while Mom took one look at the mess and shook her head.

Dad tried to save face by grabbing some half-popped kernels. “See? Perfectly edible!” he said, popping a few in his mouth. He hadn't been very convincing to begin with, and it only got worse when he spat out the popcorn moments later in disgust.

We spent the rest of the night cleaning popcorn out of every nook and cranny of that microwave.

Uno Upset

Game night in 1978 was supposed to be a friendly family affair. My brother, my parents, Grandma, and I settled in for a classic round of Uno, expecting some light-hearted fun. But nobody knew that Grandma had a hidden competitive streak that was about to make Uno feel like a high-stakes poker game.

At first, everything was calm, laughs were had, and Grandma smiled sweetly as she laid down reds and greens. But then she picked up a Draw Four card, and I swear, her whole demeanor changed. She gave a slow, devilish grin with her dentures and said, "Oh, you're in trouble now, kids."

A few rounds later, my brother was one card away from victory, so close he could taste it. But Grandma didn't even flinch. She just looked him square in the eye, and with the precision of a gunslinger, slapped down that Draw Four.

"Draw four, sonny!" she declared, a glint in her eye. My brother fumbled to pick up four new cards; his dreams of victory crumbled to the ground.

Then she turned on me, and I actually gulped. Sure enough, she laid down a Draw Two, her gaze as sharp as the cards in her hand. "Better luck next time, sweetie," she said, not an ounce of remorse in her voice.

Grandma was on a roll, ruthlessly wielding Skips, Reverses, and Wild cards like she was plotting world domination. My mom whispered, "Where did she learn to play like this?" Dad just shrugged, too busy being nullified by multiple Skip card attacks.

By the end, Grandma had annihilated every one of us. She sat back, cackling as she slapped down her penultimate card like a seasoned card shark. "Uno!" she crowed; we all stared in disbelief as she somehow got to put down her final card, too, without any opposition.

From then on, whenever we had game nights together, we’d nervously watch "Wild Card" Grandma, who would simply smirk in turn. "Who knows what cards I've got up my sleeves, hmm?"

The 1980s

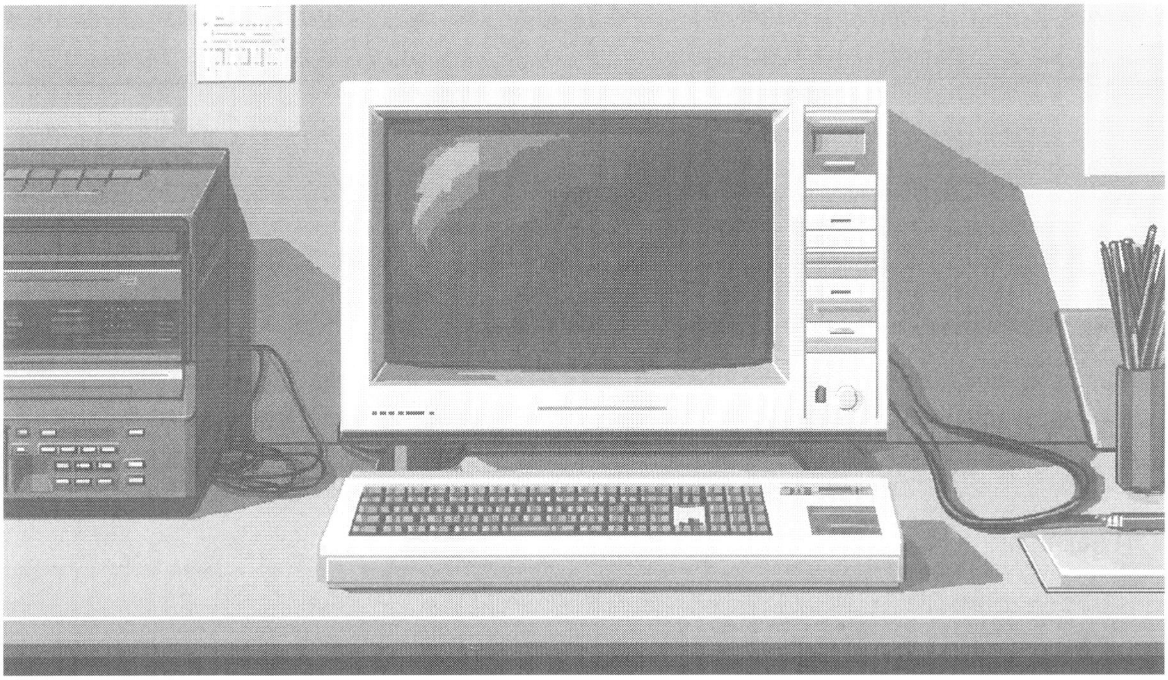

The Madonna Look

It was 1984, and my daughter Jenny was going through her Madonna phase. After watching *Like a Virgin* on MTV, she decided she had to channel her inner *Material Girl* for spirit week at school. She spent what felt like hours piecing together an outfit: fishnet gloves, an armful of bangles, a lace bow in her teased hair, layers of necklaces, and a bold amount of blush. She finished the look with a skirt over leggings and my old studded belt. She certainly looked the part of a Madonna!

As she strutted downstairs, I almost choked on my coffee. "Jenny, are you sure that's… appropriate for school?"

"It's Madonna, Mom!" she insisted, twirling dramatically. "It's the fashion now."

It was too early in the morning to argue with a 13-year-old, so I let her off, radiating confidence as she left. But just two hours later, the phone rang. It was the school principal, Mrs. Donnelly, and I could already hear the suppressed laughter in her voice.

"Mrs. Flanders," she started. "We've had… an incident with Jenny's outfit."

Apparently, Jenny's Madonna look had caused quite a stir in the halls. Boys were practically walking into lockers, girls were torn between admiration and outrage, and the teachers didn't know what to do with her. Mrs. Donnelly tried to explain to Jenny that the school had a dress code, but Jenny had stood her ground.

"Madonna says to express yourself!" Jenny had declared, causing quite the scene. "This is me!"

But Mrs. Donnelly was the school principal for good reason. Jenny was firmly sent home, fuming, with a note pinned to her jacket and a stern lecture about "school standards." When she walked through the door, looking less like a virgin and more like a wilted tulip, I had to fight to keep a straight face.

Jenny crossed her arms, pouting. “I can’t believe they don’t understand fashion.”

I chuckled, “This isn't the kind of "material" they want you to focus on at school, Jenny.”

Pac-Man Showdown

It was the summer of 1982, and Todd’s basement had become the battleground for the fiercest competition in town—the Great Pac-Man Showdown. Every Friday night, the neighborhood kids would gather around the old Pac-Man machine Todd had scored at a garage sale. The stakes were high: Whoever got the highest score each week would win the “Golden Joystick”—a spray-painted plastic joystick Todd had hot-glued to a piece of cardboard.

Frankie “Fast Hands” Jones had held the top score for three weeks running, and he was becoming downright unbearable, strutting around the basement with his mullet bouncing, bragging about his superior Pac-Man strategy.

So one night, Danny “Slices” Murphy declared he would take Frankie down, having lived on only pizza for the last few days in preparation. He got off to a smashing start, dominating the first maze as the others looked on in awe. But in the third level, he got cornered by Inky and Clyde, and died.

"You're gonna need more pizza to beat me, Slices!" Frankie chortled.

But then, Ronnie "Gummy Bear" Astley stepped up to the machine, "emergency" candy stashed down her pockets. She darted through the maze, chomping dots and dodging the ghosts like her life depended on it. Everyone was on edge, bouncing with anxious energy. Frankie stood in the corner, arms crossed, nervously chewing his gum.

When Ronnie was only 1000 points away from beating Frankie, he pulled his last trick—he slapped the side of the machine, shaking it slightly. "Hey!" the others yelled as they tugged him away. "No foul play!"

But Ronnie's resolve was unshakeable. With one final gobble, she beat Frankie's score. The basement exploded in cheers as Danny lifted her hand up like she had just won a heavyweight bout.

Frankie stormed out while Todd grinned at Ronnie. "Way to take him down a peg, Gummy Bear!" With a wink, he whispered, "And don't worry, I won't tell anyone how much you've been practicing down here in secret."

Can You Complete a Rubik's Cube?

In 1985, the craze over the Rubik's Cube had hit Jefferson University like a tidal wave. Nearly everyone had a cube, and the goal was clear: be the first to complete it. Most of them spent more time twisting it around in frustration than actually solving it, though.

One Saturday afternoon, Tyler, Jake, and Lisa gathered in Jake's college dorm for an "Ultimate Cube-Off," each determined to solve the cube faster than anyone else. Lisa was known for her concentration, Jake for his stubbornness, and Tyler liked to bend the rules when he could.

After about fifteen minutes of watching Jake contort his face as he tried different moves, Tyler grinned and handed him his finished cube. "I figured most of it out last night," he bragged. "You want to learn from a pro?"

"Finished it, huh?" Jake eyed him suspiciously. "You just learned what a Rubik's Cube was last week!"

Lisa wasn't paying attention. She was dead set on solving her cube, muttering formulas she'd memorized from a college library book. "If I just do the R-U-R', then... wait, where's the red piece supposed to go?" she groaned, tugging at her hair.

Another half hour went by, with Jake banging his cube on the table in frustration and Lisa gnashing her teeth as her cube seemed to mock her. Finally, Tyler burst out laughing, wiping away tears as Jake and Lisa glared at him.

"What's so funny, Ty?" Lisa snapped, throwing her cube down.

“Okay, okay, I confess!” Tyler said, practically doubling over. “Last night, I switched the stickers on your cubes. There’s no way you can solve them!”

The Great Nintendo Mishap

It was the summer of 1988, and 12-year-old Mike Lebowski had just gotten the coolest gift ever: a brand-new Nintendo Entertainment System. He and his friends had spent the whole day in the basement playing *Super Mario Bros.*, their thumbs sore and their eyes glued to the pixelated plumber jumping on Goombas and dodging Koopa Troopas.

That evening, Mr. Lebowski, who usually didn’t pay much attention to games, wandered into the basement just as Mario was going down a pipe. He frowned.

“Hey, isn't that Joe in the red overalls?” he asked.

“It’s Mario, Dad,” Mike replied, distractedly pressing buttons. “He's a plumber. Who's Joe?”

Mr. Lebowski’s eyebrows shot up. “I knew it! That's Joe, the plumber from next door, isn't it? Thought he’d be taller.”

Mike laughed. “No, Dad! Mario’s a video game character. He’s not real.”

Mr. Lebowski shrugged, watching as Mario went down another pipe and emerged in a different part of the level. “If he’s a plumber, why’s he running around breaking bricks and eating mushrooms? Joe sure doesn’t do that.”

Mike’s friend Tommy chimed in. “He’s saving a princess! From a dragon!”

Mr. Lebowski looked genuinely puzzled. “A plumber… saving a princess from a dragon?” He scratched his head. “Not sure Judy would let him fool about like that; she'd throw him out for sure.”

But Mr. Lebowski stuck around, even adding some commentary along the way. “Joe, watch out for that hole! Why’s he jumping on turtles? Stick to fixing pipes, Joe!”

By the time Mario lost his first life from hitting a Goomba, Mr. Lebowski was all out of sorts. “This game makes no sense!” he grumbled. “Joe should be plugging leaky sinks, not running around in a dungeon!”

Poor Joe got the worst of it, though. The next time he fixed the pipes at the Lebowskis, he was treated to a barrage of confusing jokes about princesses, dragons, and mushrooms—and left with a vague distaste for his red overalls.

Shoulder Pads

It was 1986, and Carol Dawkins was on a mission to be the most stylish mom at the PTA meeting. Inspired by her favorite show, *Dynasty*, she’d bought a blazer with shoulder pads so huge they practically had their own zip code. *Size is power*, she'd told herself in the mirror, striking her best Joan Collins pose.

As she got ready, Carol noticed one of her shoulder pads looked a little off, sagging on the right side. But she was running late, so she stuffed it back into place and hurried out the door.

At the meeting, Carol greeted her friends with her usual enthusiasm. She was in the middle of a dramatic story about PTA fundraising when she felt something shifting. Slowly, the rogue shoulder pad slipped down her arm, past her elbow, and finally settled near her chest.

But she was too deep into her story to stop. She flung her arms wide, gesturing about "upping the popcorn sales!" as the left shoulder pad started to sag, too, joining its lopsided partner. Soon, the once-powerful shoulder pads had drifted down to her chest, leaving her looking like someone feeling insecure about her figure.

In walked Principal Jenkins, the dapper, mustached heartthrob of the school district. Carol felt her heart skip a beat as she noticed him looking her way and briefly forgot her current fashion dilemma. She struck a confident pose, only to finally notice her "shoulders" were now at her stomach.

"Oh, uh..." she desperately tried to fish out the wandering pads and push them back into place.

Principal Jenkins amusedly raised an eyebrow. "Carol, bold fashion choice. Don't those usually go on the shoulders, though?"

Carol's cheeks blushed a shade of red that even the most striking makeup couldn't match. She tried to brush it off, but the PTA moms were in stitches. And for the rest of the year after, Carol would feel a twitch in her shoulders every time she saw a *Dynasty* rerun.

Walkman Workout

It was 1987, and I was determined to start a new workout routine inspired by my favorite aerobics VHS and equipped with a brand-new neon-pink Sony Walkman. I popped in my cassette tape, *Hits of the 80s*, pulled on my matching workout leg warmers, and headed out to the neighborhood park.

The warm-up went smoothly. I bopped along to *Wake Me Up Before You Go-Go*, moving my arms in sync and feeling like an exercise queen. But just as I got to the good part, the Walkman started acting up. The tape slowed down to a draggy, haunted version of George Michael, sounding like it was playing underwater.

"Not now!" I groaned, trying to get it to work again by smacking it. With a click and a whirr, it sputtered back to life, jumping into *Eye of the Tiger*. Pumped up again, I picked up the pace, striding along with newfound determination—until I realized my headphone cord had somehow tangled around my wrist.

I tried to untangle myself while keeping up my momentum and accidentally jerked the Walkman right off my belt, sending it tumbling to the ground. "No, no, no!" I gasped, trying to catch it midair. I missed, and the Walkman skidded across the sidewalk. The music blared, sputtered, and died.

Frustrated but determined, I scrambled to my feet and clipped the Walkman back on. I took a step, only to feel a pull as the headphone cord wrapped around my ankle like a lasso. One big step, and I was down again, landing with an undignified thud on my neon-pink backside.

Mortified, I glanced around, hoping nobody had seen. But across the park was my teenage nephew and his friends, who were doubled over in laughter.

I gave them a sheepish wave. I briefly thought of how my nephew had been grumpy the last couple of weeks. Maybe his laughter was worth a bruised bum and some equipment issues?

I looked at the stubbornly tangled cord, then sighed. It probably wasn't worth *this*.

Yahtzee Yell Fest

It was a quiet Friday night in 1984, and the Walker family was huddled around their dining table for their weekly Yahtzee meetup. Grandpa Earl, a man of few words but plenty of dramatic gestures, was on a hot streak. Every family member had their own lucky charms to rely on—Mr. Walker with his neon headband, Aunt Linda's rabbit-foot necklace, and newly-enrolled college student Joey Walker had his lucky set of Yahtzee dice.

The evening was humming along with the usual trash talk and occasional dice drama when Grandpa Earl did the unthinkable. On his turn, he rolled, furrowing his bushy brows as the dice clattered around the cup, then tumbled onto the table. Slowly, everyone leaned in.

There were five ones—an extremely rare *Yahtzee*.

Out of nowhere, Grandpa Earl let out a yell that would have rattled windows two towns over. "Yahtzeee!" he bellowed, launching himself out of his chair with his hands over his head like he'd just won gold at the Olympics.

But he wasn't done. Oh no. Fueled by the excitement, Grandpa Earl picked up Joey's precious dice and, with another gleeful shout, chucked them right across the room! They flew like popcorn kernels, ricocheting off walls, hitting shelves, and landing all over the place. The family erupted in laughter, and Grandma Dorothy nearly fell out of her seat from both shock and amusement.

"Those were my *lucky dice*, Grandpa!" Joey Walker shouted woefully as the family bustled around to retrieve them.

"Oh, were they?" Earl made a pretense of bending down to look for dice behind the couch and then gave up the pretense and simply sat down on the couch. "If they're so lucky, then I'm sure they'll turn up again."

They eventually found all the dice nestled in couches, under shelves, and even one that had somehow landed inside Mrs. Walker's fishbowl!

Big Hair, Bigger Problems

In 1989, big hair was everything. And no one in Oakwood University was more dedicated to hair height than Kelly Thompson. Every morning, she'd spend an hour with her arsenal: an industrial-sized can of Aqua Net, a teasing comb, and a blow dryer that roared like a jet engine. Her goal? To make her hair as high as her social status.

One Friday morning, after a particularly intense session, Kelly emerged from her bathroom with a hairdo so enormous her little brother gasped, dropping his school bag. Kelly just smirked. She knew her hairstyle was glorious, towering like a high-rise building and defying the laws of gravity.

But that day also happened to be the windiest Oakwood had seen in months. Blissfully ignorant, Kelly strutted out the front door, feeling untouchable—until she reached the bus stop and the first gust hit.

With a whoosh, her hair wobbled, then fluffed. Kelly clamped her hands down on her head, determined to protect her creation, but the wind wasn't playing fair. It whipped from all sides, sending strands of her teased masterpiece flying in every direction. Soon, Kelly looked less like a diva and more like a wind-blown tumbleweed.

She squinted against the gusts as the bus pulled up, and just as she climbed aboard, a particularly strong breeze blew her hair sideways, smacking her in the face! She stumbled into her seat, trying to salvage what was left of her 'do, only to hear snickers and comments about bird's nests while her cheeks burned.

By the time she made it to campus, Kelly's hair had collapsed entirely, one side flattened, the other half sticking out at a wild angle, like a science experiment gone wrong. She dashed to the girls' bathroom to attempt an emergency repair, but it was no use—her big hair had been well and truly blown apart.

From that day forward, she was known as "Hurricane Kelly." And somewhat true to the name, she did pay much more attention to weather forecasts!

Breakdancing Competition

It was the summer of 1986, and my wedding was in full swing. My husband and I had planned a simple reception, but our friends had other ideas. Someone brought a boombox, someone else had a *Breakin'* soundtrack tape, and before I knew it, a breakdancing competition erupted right on the dance floor.

Guests were taking turns, busting out their best moves, from the worm to the windmill. Then, just as I was catching my breath from laughing, I heard the DJ announce, "Alright, folks, give it up for... Father of the Bride!"

I whipped around in horror to see my dad, in suit and tie, stepping onto the dance floor, his grin wide as ever. He threw off his jacket, rolled up his sleeves, and looked at the boombox like it had personally challenged him.

The crowd roared with laughter and applause as Dad crouched down. Then, in true '80s dad fashion, he started with what he probably thought was the "robot"—arms stiff, jerking from side to side, his movements more mechanical than funky. The crowd ate it up.

But Dad wasn't done. Fueled by the cheers, he got down on one knee and tried to pull off the classic spin move. But his shoe caught on the dance floor, and instead of spinning, he toppled over, landing hard on his back. For a split second, there was silence as everyone worried for his safety. Then, without missing a beat, Dad goofily stuck one leg in the air and wiggled his foot, striking a pose as if he'd meant to do it all along.

Everyone burst into laughter, clapping and cheering like he'd just won a dance-off. My new husband ran over to help him up, and Dad, slightly wobbly but beaming, brushed himself off and gave a triumphant thumbs-up.

Later, my husband confided in me. "I'm not sure I'll ever be able to top that."

I patted his arm. "Don't worry, darling. I'm not sure I'll ever want you to."

Cassette Mixed Tapes

It was 1987, and my best friend Julie had just made me the ultimate mixtape. She'd carefully recorded all our favorite songs from the radio—every hit from Bon Jovi to Cyndi Lauper, complete with DJ chatter and the occasional shout-out to "KRQ 97's hottest listeners." She had decorated the cassette with neon markers and stickers and gave it to me with a solemn look in her eye.

"This is for *life moments*," she said. "Play it during only the best times."

That Friday, we took my fiancé Bruce's car for a spin for the first time (with his permission—kind of!) and blasted the tape as loud as it would go. We sang at the top of our lungs, head-banging to *Livin' on a Prayer*, lip-syncing to *Take On Me*. It was glorious.

But then we hit our favorite part: *Girls Just Wanna Have Fun*. Just as we were in full Cyndi Lauper mode, I heard a horrible grinding sound. The music warbled, slowed, and suddenly stopped. I popped open the cassette player, and there it was—the tape had unspooled, long strands of magnetic ribbon hanging out like spaghetti.

Julie screamed. "No! My mixtape!" I tried to wind it back with my finger, but it only made the mess worse.

Julie grabbed a pencil, the ultimate tool for cassette surgery. "You have to be gentle," she declared anxiously, eyes narrowed as she tried to reel the tape back in. But in her frenzied attempt, she tugged a little too hard, and suddenly, a mess of tangled tape exploded into her hands.

We sat there, staring. Julie slumped back in her seat. "All those songs...gone *forever*," she whispered a little too dramatically.

Just then, Bruce walked up to us and took in our situation with a single sympathetic glance. Then he mused, "The songs are still on the radio, ladies. Think of this as an excuse to make a new tape of them together."

He winked. "After all... Don't you girls just wanna have fun?"

Aerobics Class Challenge

In 1985, aerobics classes were the place to be, and wearing the right outfit was half the battle. So when Fiona signed up for Sheila's *Aerobic Blast* class at the local rec center, she knew she had to look the part. She showed up in a neon orange leotard, headband, and a pair of leg warmers so bright they could blind people in direct sunlight.

The moment she walked in, she saw that Sheila had brought her A-game, too, in a metallic gold leotard, coordinating wristbands, and the tallest pair of aqua-blue leg warmers Fiona had ever seen. Instantly, there was a spark of competition; Fiona just had to out-leg-warm everyone in the room. And she wasn't the only one to think so!

The music started blaring through the speakers, and Sheila led them into a series of high kicks and side lunges. Fiona kicked higher, lunged deeper, and bounced with extra pep, like her orange leg warmers were giving her superpowers. To her left, Linda in her fluorescent green leg warmers, glared at Fiona as she kicked her leg just a little higher. To her right, Mary was hopping wildly, her purple-striped leg warmers nearly slapping her in the face.

Then Sheila called for the ultimate challenge—jumping jacks as fast as they could. Fiona went all out, hopping like a pogo stick and hearing the collective slap of leg warmers in perfect synchronization. Then, to her horror, she felt something slide.

One of her beloved leg warmers had wriggled its way down to her ankle, and then: *Whoosh!* it flopped right off onto the floor. Fiona tripped over it, tumbling forward into Linda, who toppled into Mary, causing a domino effect of tangled leg warmers and neon chaos that sent their whole line to the floor.

The class erupted in laughter, Sheila loudest of all. As they were helped back up again, she couldn't resist commenting, "Your legs are looking a little *too* warm there, ladies."

Learning to Moonwalk

It was 1983, and Michael Jackson's Billie Jean had everyone trying to moonwalk, little Timmy and Jason included. As their "cool" uncle, Matt figured he could keep up. How hard could it be to slide backward?

One Saturday, he announced, "I'm going to learn to moonwalk!" Timmy and Jason exchanged a look, then burst into laughter.

"You're too old!" Jason snickered, pointing at his sensible loafers. "Your shoes aren't even cool!"

Challenge accepted. Matt kicked off his shoes, grabbed his cassette player, and popped in *Thriller*. The boys sat cross-legged on the living room carpet, arms crossed, smirking as if they were judging an Olympic competition.

Matt started with what he thought was a smooth slide. But instead of gliding backward like Michael Jackson, he looked more like he was scooting on ice—awkward and jerky. Timmy covered his mouth, trying not to laugh, while Jason helpfully suggested, "Maybe start smaller? Like, with a regular walk?"

Ignoring them, Matt bent his knees, pointed his toes, and tried again. This time, he managed to get one foot to slide—but then lost his balance, stumbled, and crashed into the coffee table. The boys were now openly giggling.

Finally, after a good half hour of attempts, Matt managed one decent slide. He turned around, arms raised like he'd just won the moonwalking championship of the world. "See? I did it!"

Timmy gave him a sympathetic smile. "Uncle Matt, that was pretty close! Maybe you should practice when no one's watching."

Determined, he kept at it, sliding back and forth in the kitchen late at night, much to his wife Harriet's amusement. By the next family gathering, he'd improved just enough to surprise the boys with a passable moonwalk. Their jaws dropped as Matt finished with a spin, hands up just like MJ.

They were so surprised that they didn't even notice when Matt had to pick up the vase he had accidentally knocked over with his spin. But Harriet did—that sort of thing didn't escape her!

There Should Be an Age Limit

In 1984, the hottest trend was parachute pants, and every kid in town wanted a pair. My little brother had saved up for weeks to get his flashy silver ones, and my friends and I rocked neon colors, convinced we looked like breakdancing legends. But no one expected Grandpa to want in on it.

It started one Saturday afternoon. We were all hanging out at my grandparents' house, showing off our moves, when Grandpa walked in, eyebrows raised. "What's with the flapping around? Those pants look like they'd fly away in a strong breeze!"

We tried explaining the magic of parachute pants, but Grandpa just scratched his chin thoughtfully. “Well, they do look comfortable,” he admitted, eyeing them. “Maybe I’ll get me a pair.”

We all laughed, but the next thing we knew, Grandpa dragged us down to the mall the next day and straight into the trendy clothing store, asking the bewildered clerk for “those flashy pants like the kids are wearing.” We tried to steer him toward regular jeans, but the stubborn old man wasn’t having it.

Minutes later, he emerged grinning from the dressing room in a pair of blindingly yellow parachute pants that looked like inflated bananas, accessorized with his usual suspenders. The sight of Grandpa in full 80s fashion glory nearly made my brother fall over laughing.

But Grandpa wasn't done. To prove he was "hip," he attempted a move he'd seen on TV, some sort of pop-and-lock. He froze, one leg in the air and arms out, in what he thought was a perfect breakdance pose.

Then, with a loud *rip*, the pants gave out. Right down the middle!

As Grandpa sheepishly waddled back to the dressing room, my brother gasped, "Maybe there should be an age limit on parachute pants!"

Grandpa just laughed and said, "Ha! If there's one thing I won't stand for, it's limits!" But Grandpa never did get another pair, though; he settled for being the legend who tried to breakdance—and broke his pants instead!

Mad Dash for Cabbage Patch Dolls

In 1983, Christmas was all about one thing: Cabbage Patch Dolls. Every kid wanted one, and every parent was on a mission. Polly Matthews was no exception. She'd heard a shipment of dolls was coming into the local department store, and she was ready.

On the day of the restock, Polly was up before dawn, armed with a thermos of coffee and the determination of a marathon runner. When she got to the store, there was a line wrapping around the building, and every parent there had the same crazed look in their eyes. These were no ordinary shoppers; they were *hunters*.

As soon as the doors opened, it was every person for themselves. Polly sprinted down the aisles, dodging shopping carts and weaving through crowds. But just as she reached the toys section, she recoiled in horror: there were only three dolls left.

Without hesitation, she lunged, grabbing the last doll on the shelf. But she wasn't the only one. A petite woman in a pink tracksuit had a death grip on the other side of the doll. They locked eyes, both refusing to let go.

"Ma'am," the woman growled, "my daughter's been dreaming of this doll for *months*."

"So has mine!" Polly shot back.

With a fierce tug-of-war battle underway, they each tried to wrestle the doll free. Nearby shoppers watched, unsure whether to intervene or cheer them on. Just as it seemed Polly was losing her grip, there was a sharp *rip*, and the arm the woman was clutching tore off from the rest of the doll.

“Alright.” She tossed the doll's limp arm at Polly's feet. “You can have it!” Then she quickly disappeared into the crowd. Victorious and panting, Polly clutched that Cabbage Patch Doll all the way home like it was gold.

When her daughter unwrapped the doll on Christmas morning, she noticed the stitches in its arm. "Mom, what happened here?"

Polly smirked. "Those are what we call battle scars, honey. And let me tell you about that battle..."

My First Plane Ride

In 1986, I boarded my very first plane, wide-eyed and ready for adventure. The moment I stepped into the cabin, it was like entering a new world. There were so many buttons, gadgets, and shiny things within reach, and I was determined to explore every single one.

I’d barely settled in my seat when I discovered the fold-out tray. Amazing! I must have flipped that tray up and down twenty times; I'm fairly sure the lady next to me sighed. Then I dug through the seat pocket and hit the jackpot: an airsickness bag (unused, thank goodness!), a set of flimsy plastic wings, a safety card with cartoon illustrations, and a complimentary deck of playing cards.

I figured they were for passengers, slipping everything into my backpack. Just then, a flight attendant came by with free headphones! She handed me a set with a smile, and I couldn't believe my luck.

As the flight continued, I discovered the armrest button that made my seat recline. I pressed it a little too fast and nearly whacked the seat behind me. Although I said sorry, I could feel the disapproving glare from behind me.

Then came the snack cart. When the flight attendant offered me a packet of peanuts, I asked for an extra one "for the road." She winked, clearly amused, and tossed one in. I added them to my growing loot bag, feeling like a pirate.

Finally, I noticed the tiny salt and pepper packets. They were adorable, so naturally, I swiped them, along with a napkin, a mini spoon, and even the little wings pin the flight attendant handed out to kids.

By the time we landed, my bag was stuffed. I proudly exited the plane, a grin on my face as I clutched my treasure, knowing I'd just scored enough souvenirs to last a lifetime.

When my fiancé helped unpack my bag later, she just stared. "Did you leave *anything* on the plane?"

I replied with a wink, "Only the seatbelt."

VCR Wars

In 1987, Steve and Diana bought a brand-new VCR—a marvel of modern technology that promised to make life easier—or so they thought. In reality, the VCR became the source of their greatest battle: programming it to record *anything*.

It started with Steve reading the manual like he was cracking a secret code. He pressed buttons, fast-forwarded, rewound, and stared at the flashing "12:00" with a furrowed brow. "It can't be this hard!" he muttered, jabbing buttons like he was playing an arcade game.

Diana smirked from the couch. "You sure you don't need my help, Steve?" she asked, her voice dripping with sarcasm. Steve's competitive spirit kicked in.

"Diana, I got this!" he said, waving her off. He continued pressing buttons, only to end up changing the TV channel instead. After an hour of trial and error, the "12:00" still blinked back at him like a taunt.

Finally, Diana had had enough. She marched over, snatched the remote, and said, "Move over, Steve. Let me show you how it's done." She studied the remote, punched in some numbers, and suddenly, it looked like she'd nailed it. She crossed her arms, smirking.

So they set the VCR to record *Dallas* that night. Or at least, Steve let Diana handle it. But the next morning, when they both rushed to the TV like it was Christmas morning, Diana pressed play, and... *static*.

They looked at each other, horrified, as the realization set in: she had recorded two hours of snow. Diana glared at Steve as if he'd messed it up somehow; Steve threw his hands up. "I didn't touch it, Diana! I swear!"

For months, this continued. They'd wrestle over the remote, take turns trying to record shows, and even call customer support (who were no help).

Eventually, a neighbor's kid came over and set it up in three minutes flat.

From that day on, even after they eventually upgraded from a VCR, they always felt a strange, uneasy sensation whenever they saw a clock showing "12:00."

Jelly Shoes Heartbreak

In the summer of 1985, I got my granddaughter Stella a pair of jelly shoes. And not just any jelly shoes—these were cherry red, glittery, and (as far as Stella was concerned) the key to becoming a true 80s fashion queen. She'd begged me for them for weeks, so when she finally slipped them on, her own eyes sparkled nearly as much as the shoes did!

Stella wore them everywhere: to the mall, the park, even around the house, just because she could. According to her, she had made her friends at school wildly jealous of them, and they felt like walking on sparkly clouds. But one day, the beloved jellies met a grim fate.

On a scorching July afternoon, Stella and I had to make a quick run to the grocery store. We were in a hurry, so she left her shoes in the back seat, thinking nothing of it. We were only inside for about twenty minutes, but when we walked back to the car, I could feel the heat radiating off the hood like an oven.

When Stella climbed into the back seat, she let out a yelp of shock. In the center of the seat was a glistening, sticky mess where her precious jelly shoes had been! The heat had melted them into a tragic, squishy puddle that looked a bit like someone had dropped cherry-flavored taffy on the seat.

Although Stella was shrieking her head off, I couldn't help feeling more amused than horrified. "Oh no, it looks like your shoes couldn't handle the heat, honey."

Stella continued to wail about how her friends would tease her about her jellies having a "meltdown." I was more worried about something else having a meltdown—or rather, some*one* else—so I eventually calmed Stella down by buying another pair, these ones a bubblegum pink.

From that day on, Stella developed a sudden taste for over-tuned air-conditioning. There were days when I had to bring a cardigan along before visiting her!

The 1990s

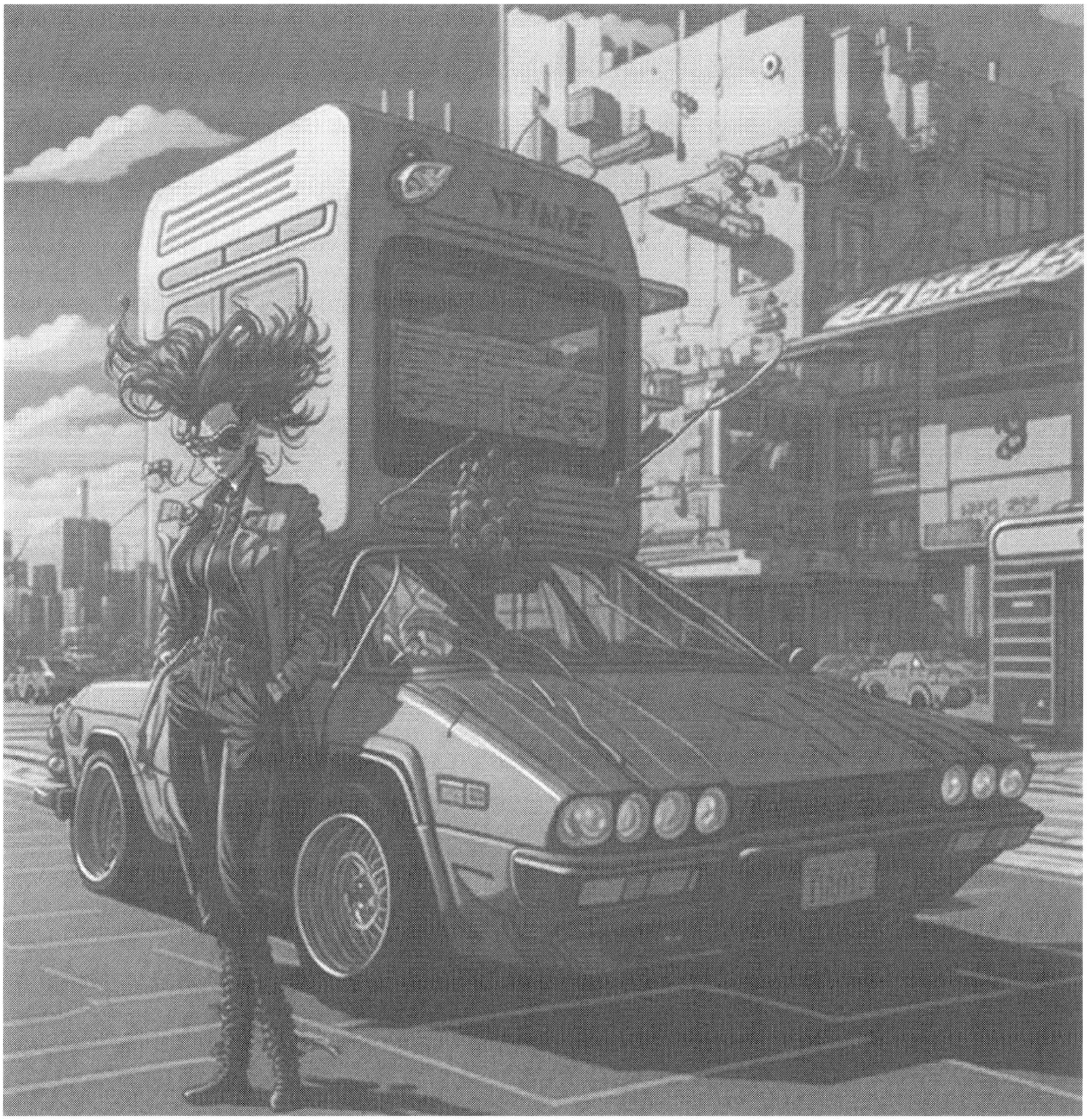

Hold On!

It was a crisp 1994 Saturday morning, and Alfred had decided to teach his neighbor's teenage kids, Jen and Mark, how to drive. Alfred's car, an ancient 1987 Buick LeSabre, looked like a tank and handled worse. But to Alfred, it was a masterpiece of reliability.

"Alright." He tapped the dashboard. "This baby has power steering, which means you shouldn't fight it—don't act like you're wrestling an alligator."

Jen sat nervously at the wheel, gripping it like she was bracing for a crash.

"Relax," Alfred said, hands poised as if catching an invisible ball. "The car can sense fear."

Jen started the car and immediately pressed the gas too hard. The Buick lurched forward, bouncing Alfred into the seatbelt.

"Easy!" Alfred barked, "We're not launching a rocket here. Think *smooth*. Be smooth."

Jen muttered an apology, barely breathing as she attempted to maneuver the Buick through a deserted parking lot. After a half-hour of cautious turns and stops, she sighed. "Okay, I think I got it!"

"Great, let's get Mark in here." Alfred waved over Jen's younger brother, who was wearing headphones and grinning like he'd just won a free pizza.

“Alright, no headphones while driving,” Alfred said, yanking the Walkman off Mark’s head. Mark sighed and buckled in, glancing in the rearview mirror and making finger guns at his reflection.

“Hey, hey,” Alfred snapped. “Eyes forward.”

Mark adjusted the mirror to look like he was complying, but the second Alfred relaxed, he slammed the gas pedal, launching the Buick with an unexpected squeal.

“Whoa! Not on my watch, Mario Andretti!” Alfred bellowed, yanking the “oh-no” handle (a.k.a. the handbrake). He fumbled with his fanny pack and pulled out a handful of Werther’s Originals. “With me, slow and steady wins the race!”

When they were done, Alfred decided to treat the kids to ice cream. While stopped at a light, Mark caught Alfred sneaking a glance at a pretty woman on the sidewalk and couldn't help calling out in his best Alfred impression: "Hey, eyes forward!"

The Y2K Countdown

It was New Year’s Eve, 1999, and the town of Mapleton was buzzing with excitement—and just a little bit of fear. People were convinced Y2K would be the end of all technology, that computers would crash, and toasters would (probably) rebel. Mapleton's community center was packed for the big dance, with a giant digital countdown clock ready to strike midnight.

In the corner, Pastor Jim had been nervously tittering about the apocalypse, clutching his Bible and casting suspicious glances at the soda machine. Mrs. Sanders, the overly enthusiastic head of the decorating committee, had distributed emergency kits to everyone. Mr. Sanders kept hungrily eyeing the cans of Vienna sausages she'd packed in the kits.

At 11:25 p.m., just as the conga line was starting to pick up, a brilliant idea struck young Willy the DJ. Willy and his friend Ollie were pranksters and had been hearing the adults drone on about Y2K for months. So they sneaked over to the countdown clock and set it ahead half an hour. Ollie snickered, "They didn't even notice!"

When midnight "struck," the dance hall erupted. People gasped as the clock flashed "00:00" and the lights flickered. Mrs. Sanders dropped her punch in horror, Pastor Jim started reciting Revelations by the soda machine, and Mr. Sanders dove under a table, clutching his sausage can like a life preserver.

"This is it!" someone shouted. "It's the *end*!"

In a frenzy, people grabbed their coats and headed for the exits when a lone voice called out, "Wait, it's only half two!" Willy and Ollie could barely breathe from giggling as they reset the clock and it blinked "11:31." The truth sank in as folks noticed the red faces of Willy and Ollie.

Mrs. Sanders laughed so hard that she snorted while Pastor Jim gave the boys a decidedly different sermon from his usual ones.

Blockbuster Bungle

It was 1997, and Lucas was a master at dodging Blockbuster late fees. Well, *mostly*. Blockbuster had cracked down on the "extend-the-rental-period-by-three-days" loophole he usually exploited, and he needed a new plan. His drinking buddies Josh and Dave were equally invested in keeping their movie nights alive without going bankrupt over late fees.

One Friday, Lucas realized their latest rental, *Space Mutants from Mars,* was a day overdue. He knew Mrs. Crenshaw, the eagle-eyed Blockbuster clerk, would catch him. She had lately developed a sixth sense for his late returns, no matter how sneaky he was.

“Fellas, we’re in trouble,” Lucas muttered, holding the bright blue VHS case like a live grenade.

Josh, the idea guy, snapped his fingers. “Easy fix! We just disguise it.”

“Disguise it?” Lucas raised an eyebrow. “It’s a *movie*, not a wanted criminal.”

“Think about it,” Josh insisted. “We put the tape in another case, something no one would rent! Like... the *Aerobics for Beginners* case—it’s been on the shelf for weeks!”

They quickly swapped the tapes, sliding *Space Mutants from Mars* into the neon pink aerobics case. Feeling like geniuses, they tried to act casual as they dropped the *Space Mutants from Mars* case into the return slot. Mrs. Crenshaw barely glanced their way, and they breathed a sigh of relief.

But then came Saturday night. Just as they settled in with popcorn and soda, the phone rang. Josh picked it up, then paled, mouthing, "It's her!"

Mrs. Crenshaw stated firmly, "Lucas, *Aerobics for Beginners* somehow found its way into the *Space Mutants* box, and the *Aerobics* case is missing. Care to explain?"

Lucas stammered, "Ah, um, maybe the space mutants... really needed some exercise?"

The next day, Mrs. Crenshaw almost cracked a smile when the *Aerobics* case was guiltily slid under the door with *Space Mutants* and a five-dollar bill inside it.

Dial-Up Drama

In 1998, getting online was an adventure for Rose Henderson. Her family's computer was an ancient beast, and its dial-up internet connection was as reliable as a secretary with short-term memory loss.

One Saturday afternoon, Rose was waiting for an important message from her friend Kelly, who was sending her a top-secret routine for maintaining healthy skin. Armed with a glass of wine, Rose sat down and double-clicked the AOL icon.

The modem screeched like a robotic cat in a blender, and she waited. And waited. But all she got was the dreaded "busy signal." Rose sighed, hit "Connect" again, and listened to the dial tone. But just as it seemed like she might actually make it online, her daughter picked up the phone downstairs.

"Hannah! Get off the phone!" Rose yelled, but it was too late—the connection cut out with a sad beep. After a few minutes, Rose heard her daughter yell up the stairs, "Did you need the phone, mom?"

Rose clenched her fists but decided to try again. She waited for Hannah's conversation to end, then clicked "Connect" one more time. The modem started its symphony of beeps and static, and this time, she actually got through! She was *online!* The familiar AOL "You've Got Mail!" voice chimed, and Rose grinned.

But before she could open her inbox, her husband yelled from the basement, "Internet's down again! Rose, are you on the phone line?"

"Honey, I'm checking my email!"

"Well, I'm trying to download updates for my weather-tracking software!" She normally didn't mind her husband's weather-tracking hobby, but now he was *hogging her bandwidth*.

Frustrated, she clicked "Disconnect" and stomped down to find him. They made a reluctant truce: ten minutes of internet each.

Finally, after what felt like hours, Rose got back online. She clicked to open Kelly's email—and waited for it to load.

When it finally appeared, it read, "Couldn't get a long enough spell at the computer. I'll send the routine tomorrow."

Fax Machine Fiasco

In 1995, my son Javier was twelve and home alone, bored and curious about the mysterious device I had brought home from work: the fax machine. The enigmatic beige box sat on our kitchen counter with its chunky buttons and a strange, alluring paper slot that simply reeked of temptation.

He'd heard rumors at school that if you sent your face through a fax machine, it would print a perfect copy of your face on the other end. So, *of course*, he wanted to find out the truth.

He flipped up the cover, carefully positioning his face over the slot, and pressed "Start." The machine whirred to life, emitting a mechanical hum that sent a chill down his spine. The light inside the scanner flickered as it dragged his face across the glass.

That was when he realized he was *stuck*.

He twisted his neck, but his cheek was suctioned onto the glass like a stubborn sticker. Meanwhile, the fax machine kept whirring, pulling his face along while making loud, stuttering beeps. He tried to pull away, but every tug felt like his skin was getting vacuum-sealed to the machine.

Just as panic set in, the door opened. My wife and I entered the scene, greeted by a curious sight: our son with his face smooshed against the fax machine while it printed a warped, stretched version of his nose across the page.

“Javier, what on Earth are you doing?” my wife shrieked.

“Research?” he mumbled, finally managing to free his face with a loud pop.

I held up the printout of Javier's squashed face, which looked more like abstract art than anything recognizable. “Well, I guess that’s one way to use a fax machine,” I chuckled.

“Did it work?” he asked, feeling his nose as though to check if it had flattened permanently.

I laughed. "Oh, the machine's functioning like it should. I'm not as sure about you, though, son!"

Baby in Waiting, Pager Not Found

It was the summer of 1996, and Benjy was nervously pacing the grocery store, clutching a half-completed shopping list while glancing at his belt every few seconds. His wife Linda was due any day now, and her doctor had given Benjy a pager to keep on him at all times for the big moment.

This was no ordinary pager. It was bright neon green, huge, and hung from his belt like a brick. Benjy thought he looked ridiculous. The grocery store clerk probably thought he was a doctor or secret agent. After all, Linda *had* snorted and called him "Secret Agent Pager" earlier.

Halfway through the cereal aisle, Benjy felt an ominous emptiness on his hip. He looked down. The pager was *gone*.

"Oh no..." he spun in place and scanned the floor like he was looking for buried treasure.

Frantically, he retraced his steps. No pager in the dairy section; none by the canned goods. He checked the freezer section and even backtracked to produce. *Nothing*. Just then, his thoughts were interrupted by a beeping sound echoing faintly somewhere nearby. It was the pager's locator tone that Linda had insisted he turn on. But where was it?

Benjy paused, trying to follow the sound. Then, to his horror, he realized it was coming from the cash register. The woman at checkout held up his pager playfully, dangling it like a lost puppy, beeping loudly for all the store to hear.

Benjy's face flushed as he grabbed the pager. "Uh, thanks. Baby on the way," he mumbled, trying to sound casual.

"Congratulations," she grinned. "You'll need to be on your toes once the little one arrives."

As he walked out, the pager went off again. Heart pounding, he looked at the message from Linda: "Where are you? Baby almost here!"

He sprinted out of the store and was halfway to the hospital when he realized he'd left the shopping in the store. Secret Agent Pager's mission was feeling more impossible by the minute!

Learning To Text

In 1999, I finally got a cell phone of my own. It was a chunky Nokia, as sleek as a brick, and my daughter Annie was beyond excited. She couldn't wait for me to try the new thing she'd heard about: text messaging. Her best friend, Sarah, was already an expert texter, so Annie arranged for me to have my first text exchange that night.

I sat down, flipping open her Nokia and staring at the buttons. *How hard can it be?* I thought. I started typing "Hi," which should've been easy. But on these old phones, each button had three or four letters, and I had to hit each one just the right number of times.

First, I needed "H" from the 4 key. But I hit it one too many times, ending up with "I." I hit *backspace*, but somehow, that erased the whole message. I tried again, slowly and carefully pressing 4 two times—finally, "H" appeared.

Next, the "I." I hit 4 three times, and miraculously, "Hi" was on the screen. Elated, I pressed *send*. A few seconds later, the phone buzzed with Sarah's reply.

Sarah: Hi Mrs. G! :)

Feeling bold, I decided to reply with "What's up?" I pressed 9 three times to get "W," then immediately lost track of the clicks, and then the buttons, accidentally sending "Wtb" instead.

Sarah: What's 'wtb'? Is that code?

I flushed, my fingers already cramping. I tried to type, "Sorry, meant to say hi!" but it came out as "Snrsx, nebmt ts scz pq!"

The phone buzzed again.

Sarah: You OK there, Mrs. G?

I took a deep breath, determined. I concentrated hard, pressing each button like I was defusing a bomb. An eternity later, I managed to send a message.

Me: Hi! Just practicing lol.

Sarah: LOL – No worries, you'll get it, Mrs. G.

Feeling victorious, I put my phone down, fingers aching. Texting was exhausting! As I settled into my armchair for a nap, I had difficulty imagining that this kind of communication would *ever* become popular.

Learning the Macarena

It was 1996, and no party, school dance, or family reunion was complete without the Macarena. Everyone seemed to know it—everyone except yours truly. I had somehow managed to dodge learning the steps, but when my cousin's wedding rolled around, I decided it was time. If everyone was doing it, how hard could it be?

I tried practicing in my bedroom the night before with the song on a cassette. The first steps seemed simple enough. Right arm out. Left arm out. Right hand to shoulder, left hand to shoulder… Except I kept getting them backward; after a few tries, I accidentally slapped myself in the face!

By the time I got to the hip movements, I was a sweaty mess, frantically trying to keep up with the song on the tape. I looked in the mirror, only to realize I was about as graceful as a dizzy chicken. "This is hopeless," I muttered.

At the wedding reception the next day, the DJ announced, "Everybody on the floor—it's time for the Macarena!" I felt a wave of panic as my entire family cheered and jumped up. My cousin Naomi nudged me, "Come on, it's easy!"

Resigned, I followed her lead... Well, I *tried* to. Right arm out, left arm out… Wait, were they clapping already? I scrambled to catch up, looking like I was trying to pat my head and rub my belly at the same time. By the time I got my arms in the right places, everyone was swiveling their hips. I swiveled his hips in the opposite direction, bumping into Aunt Ellen, who nearly toppled over.

After many failed attempts, I thought I finally had the rhythm figured out—but then the song ended, and everyone cheered.

"Hey, you were almost there! Not bad for someone with two left feet," Naomi laughed.

I wiped my brow, grinning. "Well, at least I didn't break any bones."

Aunt Ellen chipped in sardonically, "Not for lack of trying."

VHS Taping Mistakes

In 1993, Pete had a collection of VHS tapes he guarded like treasure, especially his *Star Wars* and *Indiana Jones* trilogies. But Pete wasn't very good at *labeling* said tapes, as his son Liam helped him find out the hard way.

One rainy Saturday, Liam decided to tape over an old VHS to record his new favorite TV show, *Teenage Mutant Ninja Turtles*. He figured he'd pop in a tape, hit record, and be a hero to his friends for preserving the latest episode.

The tape he grabbed from the shelf was unlabeled, so he assumed it was a blank. *Perfect*. He pressed "record" and settled in, watching the episode while it saved to the tape. After the turtles saved the day, he popped it out, proud of himself, and put it back onto the shelf.

That night, Pete announced they'd be watching *Indiana Jones and the Last Crusade*. Liam was thrilled at the prospect of seeing one of Pete's treasures on the screen—until he saw the tape Pete picked up. It looked like the one he had used that morning!

As the family settled in with popcorn, Pete dimmed the lights, Pete's wife Beth started the VHS player, and Liam chewed his nails nervously. The familiar Lucasfilm logo appeared, and Liam breathed a sigh of relief—maybe it wasn't that tape after all!

But then the screen suddenly cut to a very different scene: the Teenage Mutant Ninja Turtles zooming across New York City.

“Uh... What’s going on?” Pete squinted at the screen.

Liam’s face went pale, and he had a burning desire to disappear into the couch cushions. The Turtles were now battling their nemesis Shredder where Indy had once fought Nazis.

“Liam...” Pete began in a tone that was both baffled and heartbroken.

“I promise, I thought it was a blank tape...” his son mumbled sheepishly.

Pete sighed, staring at the screen as Raphael and Leonardo struck ninja poses. “Of all the tapes... Why not one of your mom’s aerobics tapes?"

At this point, Beth amicably tossed a cushion at Pete's face.

Walkmans Don't Run

In 1998, Alex finally got a shiny new CD Walkman for his birthday, gifted by his son's family. With his favorite *Led Zeppelin* album loaded in, he slipped on the foam-covered headphones and headed outside to meet with his jogging group.

The problem started as soon as he stepped onto the sidewalk. Alex had barely taken three steps when the Walkman jolted, and the music cut out with a harsh "*Bzzt... skip... bzzt.*" He froze, looked down, and waited for it to play again. After a second, *Communication Breakdown* started back up, smooth as ever.

"Okay, just don't move too fast," he told himself. He started walking carefully, trying to keep his stride smooth, like he was balancing a glass of water on his head. It worked – for about ten more steps. *Bzzt!* The music skipped again.

Determined, Alex tried walking slower. He moved one foot, then the other, like he was walking on hot coals. People stared, but he didn't care. The music continued, and he smiled to himself. He'd figured it out!

Then he reached the crosswalk, where a group of people he knew from the local community center were waiting. Trying to act normal, Alex picked up his pace. *Bzzt bzzt bzzt!* The Walkman turned into a skipping mess. The group noticed and laughed.

"Alex, you're into robot noises now?" one of them teased.

Alex shrugged. "It's one of those, uh, remix versions. This DJ likes to add groovy effects." He tried to take a step, but the music cut off again.

Embarrassed but undeterred, Alex came up with a new plan. He held the Walkman out in front of him like it was a delicate artifact. He walked all the way to the meetup spot that way, hands outstretched and shuffling like a mummy. When he finally made it, he'd still only heard three uninterrupted songs.

Alex sighed. "I guess that's why they're called Walkmans instead of Runmans."

The Trouble With Email

In 1997, I finally got my first email address, and it felt like a ticket to the future. I'd watched my nephew Nate typing away with his friends and even joining this mysterious thing called a "chat room." Now, I had my very own email account: *clarissa_m1961@aol.com*.

One afternoon, I logged in, my heart almost pounding with excitement. After a few clicks and lots of squinting, I finally saw it: my first email! The subject line read, "Hey Rissa!" and it was from my best friend Karen.

Hands shaking, I clicked to open it, imagining all the amazing things Karen might've written: maybe it was a joke, a secret, or plans to hang out this weekend.

But my finger slipped, and I accidentally clicked "Delete."

The email disappeared instantly. "No, no!" I gasped, frantically clicking around the screen. I looked for an "undo" button, a "retrieve email" button—anything. But it was gone, lost in... wherever it was that emails existed.

Panicking, I clicked on the *Trash* folder, but it was empty. Did the computer actually eat it? I was baffled. Emails didn’t just vanish like that! Or did they?

Nate walked in just then and raised an eyebrow. “What’s going on, Aunt Rissa?”

“I… I got my first email, and I deleted it!”

He burst out laughing. “Oh no! It was important, I'm guessing?”

“Yes! Karen sent it, and now she’ll think I didn’t care enough to write back!” I buried my face in my hands. I’d finally stepped into the future and immediately tripped on the welcome mat.

Nate smirked and patted my arm. “Don’t worry. Just email her and tell her what happened.”

I blinked. “Oh. Right.”

I sheepishly opened a new message:

Hey Karen, I accidentally deleted your email, but I totally wanted to read it! Could you resend it?

Later that night, Karen’s response popped up:

LOL, Rissa. Sure, I’ll send it again.

I wondered why she was so amused until I saw the all-important first email—it simply said:

Hi!

I couldn't help laughing too.

The Turkey That Got Away

Thanksgiving in 1995 was supposed to be perfect. My mom was coming, my sister, Mabel, was bringing her famous pie, and my husband Sven was certain that was the year he'd redefine Thanksgiving with his latest turkey recipe, which was apparently the stuff of legends.

The trouble started when he decided to fry the turkey—it was apparently all the rage. Sven borrowed his friend Jerry's fryer, set it up in the backyard, and went over his checklist. Thawed turkey? *Check*. Peanut oil? *Check*. Fire extinguisher? *Check*. I wasn't convinced, but Sven assured me that he was in complete control.

The big moment arrived. Sven put on my "Kiss the Cook" apron, grinned at us like a kid on Christmas morning, and slowly lowered the turkey into the fryer. Just as he was about to slowly drop it in, the bird slipped from his grip and plopped into the oil with a huge splash!

Oil sprayed everywhere, and before anyone could react, flames shot up from the fryer. My mom screamed, I gasped, and Sven went into full panic mode. He fumbled for the fire extinguisher, spraying foam everywhere, while Mabel tried to shoo our kids back inside.

But things got worse. Our family dog, Sparky, ran out the back door, eyes wide, and immediately fixated on the smoldering, partially cooked turkey that Sven had yanked out of the fryer. Before anyone could stop him, Sparky leaped up, grabbed the turkey by the drumstick, and bolted into the yard with it.

We all stood there, stunned, as Sparky paraded through the yard, proudly shaking his prize like he'd just won the lottery. Sven was too covered in foam to chase him, and the rest of us were doubled over with laughter. By the time we finally caught Sparky, the turkey was a total loss, covered in dog slobber and grass.

In the end, we ordered pizza, and Mabel's pie saved the day. And after that Thanksgiving, Sven never mentioned his "legendary" recipe again.

What the *%&@#& Is My Password?

In 1998, Leo was given his very first email account. It was supposed to be a big deal, a new frontier for sending messages and even joining chat rooms. But there was one problem: *passwords*. Leo could never remember them, and this time was no different.

He'd created an account last week and had chosen a password he was certain he'd remember: something unique but simple. Yet as he sat at the computer, staring at the blank "Password" box, his mind was empty. He typed in what he thought it was: *password123*. Nope. He tried again: *passWORD123!* Wrong again.

A bead of sweat appeared on his forehead. After a few more failed attempts, a new message popped up:

Account locked. Please answer your security question to reset your password.

He breathed a sigh of relief—he'd definitely remember the answer to this! But then he saw the security question:

What is your favorite food?

"Oh, no," he muttered. Leo loved food. Was it pizza that day? Or had he been in a taco phase? Was he craving lasagna?

After three wrong guesses, he was locked out again.

Frustrated, he muttered under his breath, "What the *%&@#& is my password?"

Just then, his roommate and occasional tennis buddy Herb peeked in, amused. “Language, Leo! What’s going on?”

“I can’t remember my password, and I got locked out! I need it for work.”

Herb chuckled. “Well, we could call tech support. Maybe they can reset it.”

With Herb’s help, they finally got through to tech support. After a 20-minute hold and some awkward attempts to explain the problem, they reset his account. Leo sighed in relief as he typed in his new password: *tacocat*. He was sure he would remember it since it was a palindrome.

But the next week, when he tried to log in, he’d already forgotten it. "Oh no, not again..."

After another call to tech support, Leo finally had a password he would remember: *ohnonotagain!*

Teaching Mom How to Use the Computer

It was 1997, and our family had just gotten a brand-new computer. Naturally, my 80-year-old mom wanted to learn the ropes. I, the resident “computer expert,” was recruited as her teacher. I quickly realized that patience wasn't my strong suit.

“All right, Mom. First, turn it on.”

She squinted at the monitor, pressing random keys. I leaned over. “No, the button on the tower, Mom.”

“Oh! This thing?” she asked, jabbing the power button like it might shock her. The computer whirred to life, and she clapped delightedly.

“Okay, now we’re going to open a window,” I said, clicking on the little icon to open a program.

Mom looked alarmed. “Open a window? But it’s freezing outside!”

“Not that kind of window! It’s just a program.” She nodded, clearly having no idea what “program” meant.

We managed to open a document, and I showed her the mouse. “Just move this arrow around with the mouse.”

Mom looked at the small, gray box in her hand, skeptical. “This doesn't look anything like a mouse!”

“Just move it on the mousepad, Mom.”

She began dragging it back and forth like she was sweeping crumbs off the counter. The pointer flew wildly across the screen, landing on random icons.

“Now, click there to close the window,” I said, pointing.

Mom gasped, looking horrified. “Click there? How? Do I hit it on the screen?”

I put my head in my hands. “No, just move the arrow to the cross over there, then click the mouse!”

After an eternity, the window closed. She looked triumphant. “I did it! Now, how do I turn it off?”

“Click the 'Start' button.”

She stared blankly. “To turn it off... I hit Start?”

“Yes,” I sighed. “Welcome to computers.”

Finally, she powered down the system, looking like she’d just completed an Olympic event. She gave me a big hug and said, “Thank you, honey! Next time, you can teach me to email.”

I smiled weakly, not entirely sure I could last that long.

The 2000s

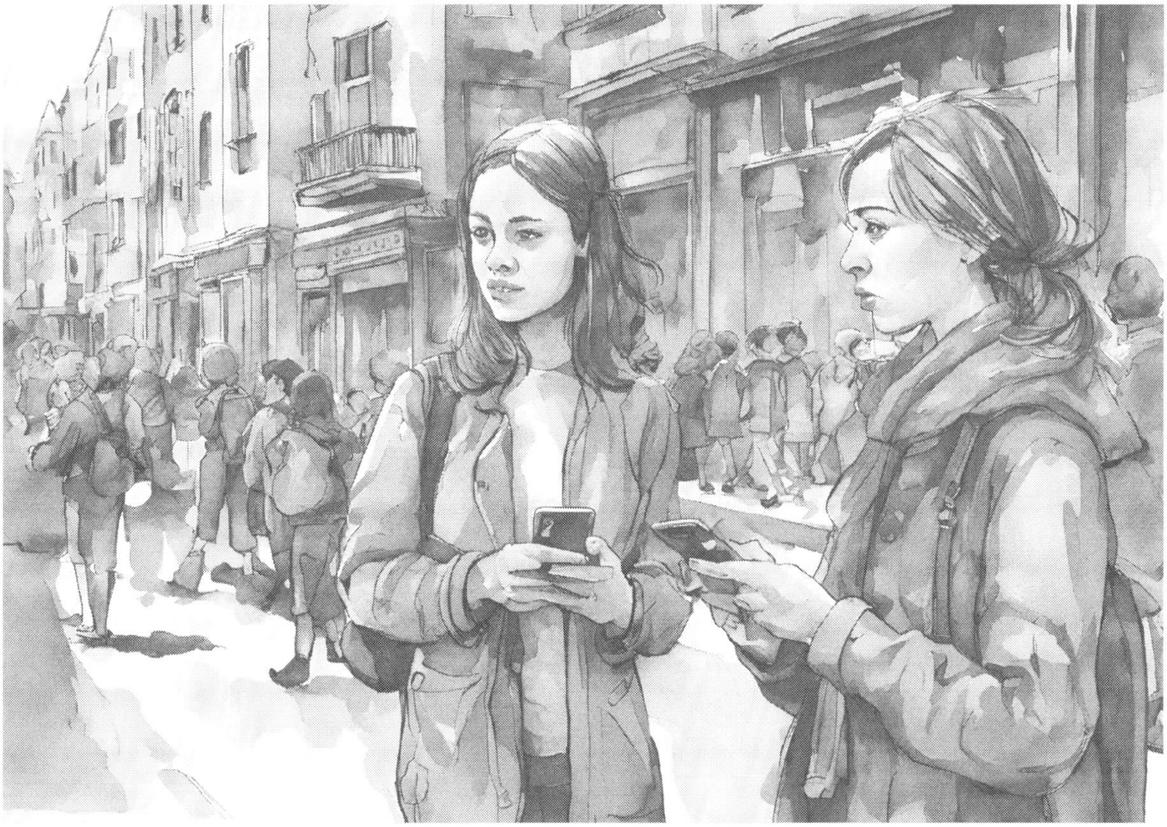

Boy Bands

It was 2003, and my daughter Kelly begged me to drive her and her friends to a concert for some "boy band" called *O-Town*. I had no idea what a boy band was; to me, it sounded like a group of kids playing backup at a talent show. "Do they play instruments?" I asked. Kelly rolled her eyes, the universal teenage sign for *you're hopeless*, and muttered, "No, Dad. They sing and dance. *Duh*."

Now, I'd grown up with *The Beatles* and *The Monkees*, so I assumed we were talking about something along those lines. But as I waited in the car outside the arena, I saw a group of scrawny teenage boys prancing by in matching metallic outfits that looked like leftovers from a failed sci-fi movie. Their hair was frosted, their shirts were unbuttoned just enough to make me uncomfortable, and they were striking poses like male models with low blood sugar.

I couldn't help myself. I yelled out the window, "Hey, are you guys a boy band?" They stopped, exchanged confused glances, and one of them yelled back, "We're *Solar Crush!* Who's asking?"

Kelly, mortified, dragged me back into the car before I could give a scathing reply about how crushed their clothes looked. "Dad, stop embarrassing me!"

"But they don't even have guitars!" I protested. "How are they a band?"

"They don't need guitars! They're hot!" Kelly hissed.

The confusion only deepened when the opening act took the stage. The *Solar Crush* boys lip-synced to pre-recorded tracks while attempting to dance in sync. It was like watching a herd of deer learning choreography. Meanwhile, the screaming teenagers acted as if Beethoven himself had descended from the heavens.

I turned to another dad in the parking lot. “So, is this what kids call music now?” He shrugged and said, “I don’t know, brother. My kid thinks my *Journey* cassettes are prehistoric.”

I sighed. “I'm feeling a little prehistoric myself.”

Trying Out for *Survivor*

It was 2004, and Greg convinced his friend Drew to try out for the reality TV show *Survivor*. Drew was a desk jockey dad with a love for snack cakes, not survival skills. Greg, however, had been hitting the gym since Y2K. "We’ll be great!” he said. “You’ve got charisma, and I’ve got biceps. We'll make a perfect duo.” It didn't occur to either of them at the time that there could only be one winner on the show.

They showed up at the casting call, which was held at some swanky mall food court. Drew looked disappointed that the setting wasn't more rugged. While Greg had his tight workout shirt on, Drew sported some trusty cargo shorts, a fishing hat, and a fanny pack stuffed with beef jerky and sunscreen—just in case he had to prove he could survive the wild right there.

The other contestants looked like they’d stepped out of a CrossFit competition. Chiseled jaws, toned arms, and confidence dripping like sweat after a good cardio session. Meanwhile, Drew was still debating whether he should have bought a pretzel from the *Auntie Anne's* they passed on the way.

The application asked about their "physical fitness routine." Drew proudly wrote "light gardening and chasing the dog when he steals socks." Greg gave him a mean look but said nothing.

Then came the interview. “So, what’s your survival strategy?” the producer asked.

“Well,” Drew began confidently, “I’ve been practicing. Just last weekend, I went two hours without AC during a power outage. Also, I once assembled an IKEA shelf without instructions. Got every nail in right where it should have gone! That’s real survival, right?”

The producer blinked. Greg buried his face in his hands.

In the end, they didn’t make it. Apparently, *Survivor* wanted folks who could run marathons and look photogenic doing it, not people who could survive a PTA meeting on three hours of sleep.

What Is a Prequel?

It was 2002, and my son Danny begged me to take him to see *Star Wars: Attack of the Clones*. My last Star Wars memory was standing in line in 1983 to see *Return of the Jedi*. Back then, there were just three movies with a simple story: rebels, bad guys, laser swords. Now, there were "prequels," and I was deeply confused.

“So, wait,” I asked Danny as we sat down with our popcorn, “this is before Luke Skywalker?”

“Yeah, it’s about his dad, Anakin,” he said, eyes rolling like a miniature Yoda, annoyed with my ignorance. “He becomes Darth Vader.”

“Well, thanks for spoiling it!” I chuckled as I got a glare in response.

The lights dimmed, and the movie started. Within ten minutes, I was hopelessly lost. Who was the tall alien with googly eyes? Why were robots fighting clones? And why was the dialogue so bad? I leaned over to Danny. “Is that dashing young man supposed to be Obi-Wan?”

Danny whispered, “It’s a prequel, Dad. Of course he’s younger here.”

“But if this is the past,” I whispered back, “why do their spaceships look shinier? And who are all these new people?”

Danny nearly shoved popcorn into my mouth to shush me up. But I couldn’t help myself. Every five minutes, I had a new question. “What’s a Sith? Is this love story important? Why are they fighting on a lava planet?”

By the time Yoda whipped out a lightsaber and started flipping around like a caffeinated frog, I gave up. “This makes no sense,” I muttered. “I liked it better when we just had the Death Star and proper space battles without fancy gymnastics.”

After the credits rolled, I couldn't help myself. "*Attack of the Clones*? More like *Attack of the Groans*, don't you think?"

I had to smile to myself as Danny responded with—what else?—a groan.

Famous Scenes From *Cars*

It was 2007, and Kenneth's five-year-old grandson, Corey, had just discovered the movie *Cars*. He was obsessed. Every conversation somehow circled back to Lightning McQueen, Radiator Springs, or—his personal favorite—Tow Mater. Kenneth, a spry 62-year-old with the flexibility of a rusty lawn chair, thereby was Corey's chosen co-star for reenactments.

One rainy Saturday, Corey dragged Kenneth to the living room stage—also known as the rug—and handed him a plastic colander. “Here, Grandpa. This is your Mater hat,” he declared. Before Kenneth could argue, Corey shoved it on his head and assigned roles. “I’m Lightning. You’re Mater. You say, ‘Dadgum!’ and do funny voices.”

“Dadgum?” Kenneth repeated skeptically.

“Louder!” Corey insisted, spinning in circles.

So there Kenneth was, a retired accountant, shouting “Dadgum!” while pretending to be a rusty tow truck. Corey zoomed around the couch, screeching tire noises and narrating his every move. “I’m going to win the Piston Cup! Vroom! Grandpa, you have to be my crew chief now!”

“Sure, champ. What do I do?”

“Yell at me! Say, ‘Faster, Lightning!’”

Kenneth obliged, doing his best impression of a NASCAR commentator. “Faster, Lightning! You’re burning rubber!”

“No, no, no!” Corey groaned, stomping his foot. “You’re not yelling enough! Be like Doc Hudson!”

Not wanting to disappoint, Kenneth cranked up the volume. “FASTER, LIGHTNING! PUSH IT TO THE LIMIT!”

Corey gave him a thumbs up. “Perfect!”

Things escalated quickly. Soon, Kenneth was lying on the floor pretending to be a crashed McQueen. Corey directed him to groan dramatically, then miraculously "get fixed" with a tire pump that was actually a flashlight—another actor thrust into a role without much say in the matter. But Kenneth delivered an Oscar-worthy performance, at least from his perspective; Corey didn't even know what the Oscars were.

By the end, though, Kenneth was exhausted, and Corey declared, “Grandpa, that was awesome. Tomorrow, we’ll do the tractor-tipping scene!”

“Can’t wait,” Kenneth drawled, already dreading the looming "tractor" role.

Swooning Over Denzel Washington and Julia Roberts

It was 2002, and Friday night movies had become an institution for Sid and Carla Palmer. That night’s pick? *The Pelican Brief*. Sid rolled his eyes when he saw the DVD cover.

“Denzel Washington and Julia Roberts,” he dramatically held the case like it was a romance novel. “I suppose I’m going to spend the next two hours hearing about how ‘perfect’ they are.”

Carla smirked. “Sid, Denzel isn’t just perfect—he’s flawless. And Julia? America’s sweetheart! Have you seen that smile?”

“Oh, please,” Sid scoffed. “We both know Julia's smile isn't why you picked this movie.”

“Correct,” Carla replied. “If Denzel showed up at this door right now and asked me to run away with him, you’d have to pack my bags.”

Sid narrowed his eyes. “Well, if Julia Roberts asked me to join *her* on a European yacht trip, I’d be gone faster than you could say *Pretty Woman*.”

“You? On a yacht with *Julia*? She’d need Dramamine after five minutes of your fishing stories,” she teased.

“And Denzel wouldn’t last ten seconds with your inability to decide where to order takeout,” he shot back while starting the movie.

As Denzel raced through a suspenseful scene, Carla sighed. “Look at him. Smart, brave, noble. Why can’t you be more like that?”

Sid waved a chip. “He’s got a script, Carla. Give me a team of writers, and I’d be saving the day, too.”

Later, when Julia charmed her way past some bad guys, Sid smiled. “That woman can handle just about anything. Why don’t you ever solve mysteries with that kind of grace?”

“Because I’m too busy cleaning up your 'mysteries,' like the socks you leave all over the house,” Carla retorted.

By the time the credits rolled, they were in hysterics, trading ridiculous “Denzel would” and “Julia could” scenarios.

“Truth is,” Sid finally said, “they’re great, but I’ll stick with you. You’re my favorite co-star.”

Carla grinned. “Same here, Sid."

Then she chuckled. "But *if* Denzel calls, you’re still packing my bags.”

Low-Rise Jeans

It was 2003, and low-rise jeans had officially taken over the world. Britney Spears wore them. Christina Aguilera wore them. Sixteen-year-old Jenna Farrell practically lived in them. "Mom, they're iconic," she'd say, strutting around like she was on a red carpet while Mr. Farrell muttered from the couch, "They're one sneeze away from disaster."

One afternoon, Jenna came home with a new pair. "You should try these, Mom," she teased. "They're making a comeback for all ages."

Mrs. Farrell laughed. "Jenna, I'm forty-three. My days of exposing belly buttons are long gone."

"Come on," she said, grinning. "YOLO, Mom."

And so, in the privacy of her bedroom, Mrs. Farrell attempted to squeeze into a pair of jeans designed for someone who didn't remember the days of rotary phones. She got them on—barely—and stood up. The jeans slid so low that Mrs. Farrell wasn't sure if she was wearing them or if they were wearing her.

As she shuffled out and into the living room, Mr. Farrell looked up from the newspaper and choked on his coffee. "Sabrina, what is... why... are those pants or a suggestion?"

"They're fashionable!" she snapped, tugging them up in a futile attempt to protect her dignity.

Just then, Jenna burst into the room. "Mom, you're rocking them!" she shrieked with laughter. "You look so Y2K!"

"What's Y2K? I thought these were... YOLO."

"It means young and cool!" Jenna chirped.

Emboldened by her encouragement, Mrs. Farrell decided to wear them later that day to pick up Jenna from soccer practice. But as she leaned into the car to grab her water bottle, the jeans betrayed her. There was a *rrrip*, followed by the unmistakable breeze of humiliation. Jenna gasped. "Mom, your underwear!"

Needless to say, the low-rise experiment ended that day, and Mrs. Farrell returned to mom jeans. But every so often, Mr. Farrell would whisper, "YOLO, Sabrina," and they'd both dissolve into fits of laughter, to Jenna's utter confusion.

Crimped Hair Fiasco

It was 2001, and Emma was graduating from high school, so she asked her favorite aunt, Linda, to come to her graduation party looking "fabulous." At

53, Linda's definition of fabulous was a pair of nice slacks and some fresh lipstick. Emma, however, had other ideas.

“Aunt Linda, let me do your hair!” she exclaimed.

Emma had a crimping iron. Aunt Linda had always thought of those things as waffle makers for the hair. She hadn’t seen one since 1987, but Emma swore, “Crimping is back!”

“Oh, I don’t know,” Linda hesitated, patting her reliable helmet of hairspray.

“Come on,” Emma begged. “You’ll look so Y2K chic!”

Linda didn’t know what Y2K chic was, but she had to cave in the face of her favorite niece. So Emma dragged her into the bathroom and got to work. The crimping iron sizzled like a campfire as she clamped Linda's hair, section by section. The smell of burning hair was mildly concerning, but Emma reassured, “It’s supposed to smell like that. It means it’s working.”

When Emma finally spun her around to face the mirror, Linda gasped. She looked like she’d stuck her head in a toaster. The once-smooth bob was now a puffball of zig-zag chaos. “What do you think?” Emma asked, beaming.

“I think I look like Einstein's long-lost sister,” Linda said, wide-eyed.

Emma laughed and declared, “You look fabulous!” before ushering her aunt into the party.

The reactions were... memorable. Linda's husband, Jim, stared at her like she'd grown a second head. "What happened to your hair?" he asked, trying not to laugh.

"It's crimped," Linda said defensively, as if that explained everything.

"You look electrifying," he replied, smirking.

By the time Linda left the party, the crimping had relaxed into something resembling "frizz on steroids." The next day, she spent two hours trying to brush it out, which resulted in a hairstyle best described as "exploded tumbleweed."

Shopping for a Polly Pocket

It was 2005, and Isabelle was on a mission to find the perfect birthday gift for her niece, Lily. She'd been begging for the newest Polly Pocket playset, and Isabelle aimed to deliver. Her father, Grandpa Joe, strangely decided to tag along, claiming he "wanted to help."

"Polly Pocket, huh?" he said, climbing into Isabelle's car. "Sounds like a clothing store for little girls. What is it—tiny jeans and shirts?"

"No, Dad," she explained. "It's a doll that comes with tiny accessories and a playset."

He grunted. “Tiny clothes still sound like a choking hazard. Back in my day, we gave kids marbles, and they figured it out.”

We arrived at the toy store, and Isabelle headed straight to the Polly Pocket aisle. Grandpa Joe, however, wandered off, grumbling something about how he would find "a proper shirt with pockets.”

Five minutes later, Isabelle found him by the clearance rack in the toddler clothing section. “Look at this!” he said, holding up a sparkly pink jacket with actual tiny pockets. “This has *gotta* be one of them Polly Pocket things. What else would it be?”

“Dad,” Isabelle sighed, “we’re looking for toys, not a bedazzled wardrobe for a four-year-old.”

He looked unconvinced. “Why’d they name it Polly Pocket if it doesn’t have pockets?” He stuffed the jacket back on the rack and followed her, muttering about how toy names used to make sense.

When they finally found the Polly Pocket aisle, he picked up a doll with a tiny beach set. “*This* is it? This isn’t a pocket. It’s a speck!”

“That’s the point,” Isabelle said. “It’s small and portable.”

He squinted at the doll’s microscopic sandals and purse. “Portable? You mean impossible to find when your kid drops it in the car. Bet they make their money selling replacements." Isabelle had to almost drag him out before he launched into a full-blown rant about toys getting sucked up the vacuum.

Amazon Shopping

It was 2006, and my son, Kevin, had finally convinced me to try the new-fangled online shopping thing called *Amazon*. "It's so easy, Mom," he said. "You'll love it. No more lugging bags around the mall." I was skeptical, but my knees *had* been complaining recently, so I decided to give it a whirl.

I settled at the computer with my reading glasses perched on my nose and a cup of tea nearby. My mission: to order a set of baking pans for the upcoming church fundraiser. Easy, right?

Kevin had shown me the basics: search, click, and buy. But after finding the perfect pans (non-stick with bonus cookie cutters!), I hit "Place Order," and nothing happened. I clicked again. Still nothing. Frustrated, I clicked a few more times, muttering, "Come on, you stupid rainforest, work your magic."

The screen finally refreshed, confirming my purchase. Feeling triumphant, I went to bed, proud of my tech-savvy accomplishment.

Three days later, a UPS truck pulled into my driveway. The driver opened the back, revealing an alarming number of boxes. "Mrs. Reynolds?" he asked, looking as confused as I felt.

"Yes?"

"Got twelve packages for you."

"*Twelve?!*" I squeaked.

Apparently, every frustrated click I made had resulted in a bunch of extra orders. I now owned not one, but *twelve* identical sets of baking pans. My garage looked like a bake sale explosion.

When Kevin stopped by later, he burst out laughing. "Mom, didn't you notice the confirmation emails?"

"Emails?" I blinked. "You didn't tell me about emails!"

"Mom," he said, wiping tears of laughter, "you've got enough pans to bake cookies for the entire state."

The next Sunday, having recovered from my online shenanigans, I hauled a stack of boxes to church and good-humoredly handed them out like Oprah. "You get a pan! And you get a pan! Everybody gets a pan!"

Setting up a Facebook Account

It was 2008, and my teenage daughter, Chloe, decided it was time for me to "get with the times" and set up a Facebook account. "Everyone's on it, Dad," she said, her thumbs flying over her phone. "You can share pictures, reconnect with old friends, and... well, stalk people, I guess, but in a totally normal way!"

"Is that what the youth do nowadays?" I asked dryly, adjusting my reading glasses. "Fine, let's do this."

Chloe plopped me in front of the computer, and the chaos began. "Okay, first we need a profile picture," she said.

I grabbed a framed photo of me holding a cake at my 40th birthday party. "This one's nice."

"Dad, no one takes pictures of pictures. I'll use my phone to scan it."

"I don't even know what that means, but okay."

Next came the bio. "What should I write?" I asked.

"Just a few lines about yourself."

After some deliberation, I typed, Dad of one, construction site surveyor, barbeque expert, occasional beer drinker. Chloe rolled her eyes. "That's lame."

"What's wrong with it?" I protested.

"Facebook isn't LinkedIn, Dad. No one cares about your construction sites."

Once we'd settled on a shorter, extremely uninspired bio (Life is short, eat dessert first), Chloe showed me how to add friends. She found my old high school flame, Melania, and sent her a friend request. Within minutes, Melania accepted, and I gasped. “Dear god, Melania still looks the same!”

“Wait until you see what she’s posting,” Chloe said, smirking.

Soon, I was scrolling like a pro, marveling at Melania’s yoga poses and discovering the fine art of poking people. I’d poked half my address book before Chloe snatched the mouse from me. “Dad, that’s weird. Stop poking everyone.”

“What’s the point of poking if I can’t poke?”

“You’re going to embarrass me.”

By the end of the day, I had three friends, a blurry cake photo, and a liking for Melania once again—or whatever it's called when you "like" all the things on someone's Facebook page.

Getting My First iPhone

It was 2007, and Lauren's husband Eduardo burst through the door waving a box like he’d just discovered fire. “Behold!” he declared. “The iPhone!”

Lauren squinted at the sleek black rectangle. “Looks like a fancy coaster.”

"You don't get it, Lauren," he said, already unboxing it like a kid on Christmas morning. "It's not just a phone. It's that, an iPod, and a web browser, all in one!"

"So... It's a really expensive way to check email?" Lauren teased. "My flip phone does that, too. And it's indestructible. Bet your iPhone isn't."

Eduardo ignored her, already mesmerized by the shiny touchscreen. "Look, Lauren. You can scroll by swiping your finger."

She leaned over. "How are you supposed to press buttons with no buttons?"

"No buttons is the point! It's revolutionary!"

Two hours later, she found him on the couch, still swiping. "Eduardo, why are you staring at Google Maps?"

"Because," he said dramatically, "I can zoom in. With my fingers!" He demonstrated the pinch-and-expand motion like he'd invented it.

"That's great, honey. But can it play Snake?"

"Lauren," he said, horrified, "the iPhone has *apps*. You don't even know what that means yet."

He proudly played her a song on the built-in iPod. "Crystal clear sound!"

"Wonderful. But my iPod Shuffle does the same thing, and it clips to my belt."

At dinner, Eduardo used the iPhone's browser to look up trivia about spaghetti. "See? No need for a computer!" he announced.

"Fascinating," Lauren deadpanned. "How many spaghetti facts do you need daily?"

Later that week, though, Lauren used the iPhone out of curiosity to check movie times and found a nearby pizza place, all in a few swipes. In less than a month, she got an iPhone of her own—but kept it a secret from Eduardo. She was sure he would never let her live it down if he found out!

Conclusion

We welcome and encourage your feedback and a review. Scan the code below, or log on to: *MitchellBradfordPublishing.pubsitepro.com*.

Find more of our increasing list of mind exercises and activity books on our website!

About The Author

Mitchell Bradford Publishing is both a publisher and a pen name for a group of talented writers with a vast array of experiences and circumstances. Their love of life and engaging people in stories, activities and puzzles is infectious. The team's desire to entertain, educate, and keep minds active is evident as they create books for seniors through toddlers, drawing on their backgrounds as parents, entrepreneurs, athletes, caregivers, social workers, educators, and world travelers. Their diverse cultures and ages bring an eclectic range of interests to their books and discussions over coffee.

We are excited to add to our growing list of publications and authors.

Check us out at: *MitchellBradfordPublishing.pubsitepro.com*

Mitchell Bradford Publishing

Image References

AberrantRealities. (May 25, 2024) *Retro old school vibes* [Image]. Pixabay. https://pixabay.com/illustrations/retro-old-school-vibes-happy-8782064/

AI-Hobby-Kunst. (February 12, 2024) *Ai Generated American Diner Retro* [Image]. Pixabay. https://pixabay.com/illustrations/ai-generated-american-diner-retro-8568804/

geralt. (September 7, 2023) *Ai Generated People Street* [Image]. Pixabay. https://pixabay.com/illustrations/ai-generated-people-street-phone-8239493/

Hey-Judas. (November 13, 2023) *Ai Generated Hippies Guitarist* [Image]. Pixabay. https://pixabay.com/illustrations/ai-generated-hippies-guitarist-8379600/

JulieZimmi2. (August 21, 2023) *Ai Generated Colorful Car* [Image]. Pixabay. https://pixabay.com/illustrations/ai-generated-colorful-car-woman-8201082/

PublicDomainPictures. (April 4, 2014) *Poster Vintage Antique* [Image]. Pixabay. https://pixabay.com/illustrations/poster-vintage-antique-war-316690/

Vilkasss. (October 28, 2024) *Ai Generated Retro Computer* [Image]. Pixabay. https://pixabay.com/illustrations/ai-generated-retro-computer-90s-9151068/

Made in United States
Troutdale, OR
03/21/2025

29941321R00111